Dr. Pierre

Optimal Physiology For Life

Pierre Cloutier, MD

"Add years to your life,
and life to your years."

"The cause of disease is
never a lack of medication."

Dr. Pierre

Optimal
Physiology
For Life

Evolution In Medicine

Pierre Cloutier, MD

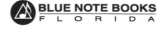
BLUE NOTE BOOKS
F L O R I D A

First Printing
Published by Blue Note Books
Cocoa Beach, Florida
1-800-624-0401

www.bluenotebooks.com

Library of Congress Control Number: 2001012345
ISBN-13: 978-0-9855562-4-2
First U.S. Edition 2012

Cover Design: Paul Maluccio

Printed in the United States of America

Contents

Introduction   11

Chapter 1
Vitamin D   13

Chapter 2
Dairy Products   21

Chapter 3
Insulin   23

Chapter 4
Medications, Drugs,   27
Supplements, Pills and Hormones

Chapter 5
Sugar   33

Chapter 6
Cholesterol   39

Chapter 7
Diabetes (Type 2)   45

Chapter 8
High Blood Pressure   51

Chapter 9
What To Eat   57

Chapter 10
Kids' Menus   63

Chapter 11
Cooking of Food   67
(The Missing Link in Nutrition)

Chapter 12
Food Allergy   71

Chapter 13
Gout   77

Chapter 14
Restless Leg Syndrome   81

Chapter 15
Actual Medicine   85

Chapter 16
Hormones (Endocrine)   89

Chapter 17
Thyroid Hormone   93

Chapter 18
Melatonin Hormone   99

Chapter 19
Growth Hormone   103

Chapter 20
Cortisone   109

Chapter 21
DHEA   117

Chapter 22
Pregnenolone   121

Chapter 23
Aldosterone   123

Contents

Chapter 24
Estrogen   125

Chapter 25
Progesterone For Women   131

Chapter 26
Testosterone and Women   137

Chapter 27
Testosterone In Men   141

Chapter 28
Contraception For Women   149

Chapter 29
Hormones and Fear of Cancer   153

Chapter 30
A Star of Medical Research   161

Chapter 31
Carnosine (An Outstanding Supplement)   169

Chapter 32
Vitamin A   173

Chapter 33
Iron (too much) - Hemochromatosis   179

Chapter 34
Omega-3 (fatty acids)   183

Chapter 35
Vitamin B-12 Deficiency   189
(More common than you think)

Chapter 36
Iodine (Deficiency)   193

Chapter 37
Dementia/Cognitive Decline/Alzheimer's   197

Chapter 38
Breast Cancer   205

Chapter 39
Bioidentical Hormones   213

Chapter 40
Fibromyalgia   221

Chapter 41
Chronic Fatigue (Syndrome)   225

Chapter 42
Addictions   231

Chapter 43
Depression   237

Chapter 44
Skin Cancer & Sunscreen   245

Chapter 45
Cardio-Vascular Disease   249
(Arteriosclerosis)

Chapter 46
Obesity   257

Chapter 47
Alcoholism   263

Chapter 48
Psoriasis   267

Contents

Chapter 49
Head Trauma   271
Traumatic Brain Injury

Chapter 50
Fatty Liver   275
Nonalcoholic Fatty Liver Disease

Chapter 51
Osteoporosis (weak bones)   279

Chapter 52
Migraines   287

Chapter 53
Conclusion   291

References   295

Index   303

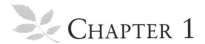

CHAPTER 1

Vitamin D
A Steroid Hormone

If all the people in America had the right amount of vitamin D (vitamin 25 OH D-measured in a blood test, optimal result is about 70 ng/ml or 200 nmol/l), health care costs would be slashed by 30%. In studies, vitamin D supplements reduced breast cancer by 50% to 75%, reduced prostate cancer by 50%, and reduced colon cancer by 50%. It is also good for your mood, the immune system and bones.

In the town where I work, Schefferville, Northern Quebec, our optometrist (vision specialist) told me she saw many children who have myopia (cannot see far), while their parents and grandparents enjoyed normal vision. Myopia is supposed to run in families, but it was new in those families, so something must have happened to change that.

I started to research the subject of myopia and found a study done in Russia where they gave vitamin D3 supplements to pregnant women and it did reduce the myopia by 80% in their newborn babies.

In the past, the Amerindians of the north (Indians native to Canada) were living in tents. They were outside most of the time. Their faces were exposed to the sun for some five hours per day, giving pregnant mothers enough vitamin D that the eyes of their babies would develop normally. Now, the Amerindians live in houses and drive pickups. I did measure their vitamin D level and they were all low. So now I give them vitamin D3 supplements.

When you have a cold or influenza, low vitamin D in your body will make the symptoms a lot worse. Remember the panic surrounding the H1N1 influenza? The vaccination can protect you from the H1N1, but vitamin D supplements in the right dosage would protect you from all kinds of influenza, cancer, depression (low mood), and weak bones.

You get vitamin D through sun exposure. The sun's rays provoke a chemical reaction with the cholesterol close to the surface of the skin, which transforms the cholesterol into vitamin D. Black-skinned people need five times more sun exposure to get the same amount of vitamin D as those with white skin.

We are made to play in the sun. With our busy lifestyles, we reduce sun exposure and we have been told that the sun's rays may cause skin cancer. Could we take vitamin D3 supplements and not expose ourselves to the sun in order to avoid skin cancer? Let's talk about it.

Since the popular use of sun block lotions, there has been no reduction in skin cancer. The idea was good but it does not work! To expose our skin to the sun must be good, since we need the vitamin D. So, how can we expose our skin to the sun and at the same time reduce the risk of cancer?

First, do not use sunscreen lotions all the time. The chemical they contain can react with the sun's rays and become toxic. Use zinc-based sun block instead on the face or other places that cannot avoid the sun and for other parts of the body use clothing. For most people who have enough vitamin D, the skin will not burn in the sun if exposure is less than one hour. So, most people do not need protection if sun exposure is less than one hour. It is also important to know that if you use sunscreen lotion, a lot less vitamin D will be made in the skin during sun exposure.

To summarize, exposing your skin to the sun without protection for up to one hour, is good! For longer exposure, use sun block (zinc-based) and clothing. Lack of vitamin D will make your skin burn faster. So, be sure to take vitamin D supplements before going in the sun. Cancers are known to start when a sunburn happens in a cell with low vitamin D. So do not expose yourself long enough to get burned.

Vitamin D is a hormone because it is made inside our body where it regulates 2,000 genes. So, it does a lot more than we think—calcium absorption, inflammation, etc. Vitamin D is a steroid hormone because it is made from cholesterol. All steroid hormones in our body are made from cholesterol. We can look at the derivation of the word: chole-sterol–sterol–steroid. You see the connection?

Is cholesterol bad for you? It is the building blocks of your steroid hormones!

A Story:

In Canada, a group from the University of Calgary made a study on seasonal variations of vitamin D and cholesterol. They found that, during the winter, when the vitamin D level is lowest, the cholesterol is highest. Interesting to see the body reacting to a low level of a steroid hormone (vitamin D) by increasing the level of the building blocks (cholesterol) that will be more elevated in the skin. When the sun's rays hit the skin, there will be more chances that vitamin D will be made.

So, what I am telling you is, when cholesterol increases in your blood, it is because your body is trying to repair something. Cholesterol will increase in reaction to low vitamin D and will increase in reaction to a low level of any of your steroid hormones (testosterone, estradiol, DHEA, pregnenolone, and cortisone).

Maintaining your steroid hormones at their right levels is needed in order to have a perfect level of cholesterol.

When your cholesterol is high, it is probably because one or many of your steroid hormones is low. By taking a supplement of those hormones to bring them to their optimal level, the cholesterol in your blood will come back to its normal level. This says that your steroid hormones are in the correct range now. That is the basic physiology of steroid hormones.

Also, when your steroid hormones are low, you have symptoms such as low libido, low mood, low muscle mass, low energy, etc. When you take a supplement of those hormones, you will correct those symptoms and at the same time correct the cholesterol.

It would be great to repair the glands that make these hormones, but the enzymatic process may be damaged in this condition by pesticides, heavy metals, hormone mimickers (chemicals), and other causes, and cannot be repaired at this time.

One thing that can be done is to reduce the loss of steroid hormones in the stools. This is because steroid hormones have a hepatic-enteric circulation. This means they are evacuated by the liver in the bile and, depending on what happens with the digestion, they may be completely evacuated or reabsorbed by the intestines, coming back into the blood.

Fibers from cereals (flour, wheat, whole grain) have a tendency to bind to the steroid hormones and evacuate them in the stools. This means you lose them! Fibers from fruits and vegetables do not bind to the steroid hormones in the intestines and those hormones are reabsorbed in the blood for a second usage. You lose less in the stools, which means you have more. Again, if you want to have more steroid hormones, stop eating whole grain cereals. For fiber, eat fruits and vegetables.

Our genes are 40,000 years old and humans just started to eat cereals (flour) in the last 10,000 years. For the first 30,000 years, humans never did eat cereals. That was the Paleolithic era with the Paleolithic diet (hunter gatherer).

The Paleolithic diet consists of fish, chicken, meat, eggs, fruits, vegetables, and nuts. Add to it good fats, such as olive oil, fish oil, some animal fat (organic) and you are all set to enjoy your food and life.

Animal fat should be cooked at low temperatures— boiled or in a crock pot. It is the cooking at high temperatures, grilled or fried, that gave animal fat a bad reputation because high-temperature cooking transforms the good animal fat to bad trans fat, which is very inflammatory.

Remember, cereals and dairy have been introduced in the human diet late in history. The protein that they contain, the GLUTEN in the cereals, the CASEIN in dairy, can cause inflammation in anyone who is sensitive. Humans are the only animals who eat dairy after the babies' nursing age. More in the next chapter.

If you are going to take the maximum recommended, because you do not get enough sun exposure or your skin is black, I recommend you have vitamin 25 OH D levels tested in your blood to be sure it is in the safe range (50-80ng/ml), (75-250 nmol/L).

On a safety note, those who should not take vitamin

D in high dosages are the patients who have sarcoidosis or tuberculosis, because they have faulty metabolism of vitamin D.

Symptoms of intoxication to vitamin D can happen if you take more than 50,000 international units per day for more than six months. Those symptoms include hypercalcemia (high calcium), nausea, and vomiting. You see vitamin D is quite safe. I have never seen intoxication from vitamin D at the recommended dosage.

Note: When you are going to take vitamin D3 supplements at the dosage recommended, you will not need a calcium supplement. This is because a study on dosage of calcium supplementation in women showed

Recommended Vitamin D3 Supplements	
0-6 months of age:	400-1000 iu per day
6 months-2 years:	1000-2000 iu per day
2 years-12 years:	2000-5000 iu per day
Over 12 years:	5000-10,000 iu per day
(iu = international units)	

those women were all low in vitamin D. They were not absorbing the calcium properly, so 1500 mg of calcium was needed to have enough (in that study).

When your body has enough vitamin D, you will absorb the calcium you eat and 500 mg of calcium per day is enough. Do not take calcium supplements if your normal diet includes green vegetables and salads as they contain enough calcium. You do not need dairy products either.

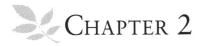 CHAPTER 2

Dairy Products

Humans are the only animals who eat dairy after they are weaned. Dairy products are a big industry, but there is no scientific evidence that dairy is good for you. Studies show that women who drink milk have more osteoporosis (weak bones) than women who do not drink milk.[*]

Milk contains calcium, but it is not absorbed well by the body. When you take vitamin D supplements, you do not need calcium supplements. Milk contains a lot of sugar (lactose) and many people do not absorb it well. Proteins (casein) in the milk may be allergenic for some people and difficult to digest because the enzymes needed to digest the casein may be damaged by heavy metals. The animal fat in the milk is not that bad if the cow is organically raised.

All the fat-soluble toxins go into the fat—pesticides, you name it. So as I said, from the nutritional point of view, dairy products are "so-so," meaning they can be inflammatory for some people.

If you have breast sensitivity, migraines, eczema, intestinal problems or are just not feeling well, I would try to avoid dairy for a month. If there is improvement, good. Stop dairy for good. If there is no change, then dairy was not the cause of your problems.

* Feskanich D. Willett WC, Colditz GA, Calcium, vitamn D, milk consumption and hip fractures, a prospective study among postmenopausal women, AM J Clin Nuir 2003;77;504-511.

* Kanis JA, Johansson H. Oden A. et al. A Meta-analysis of milk intake and fracture risk: low utility for case finding. Osteoporosis Int 2005:16:799-804.

* Weinsier RI, Krumdiek, CL. Dairy foods and bone health: examination of the evidence. Am J Clin Nutr 2000;72;681-689.

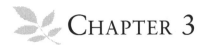 CHAPTER 3

Insulin
The Aging Hormone

Insulin is a hormone made in the pancreas and secreted into the blood, according to the level of sugar in the blood. When insulin is high, because you eat sugar, it provokes an inflammatory state. It is very bad for you! It can cause high blood pressure and inflammation of the lining of your blood vessels (endothelium), which can lead to heart attacks and strokes plus promote cancer. After awhile, high insulin also causes low blood sugar and sugar craving that leads to obesity. You get the picture.

So, if you keep your insulin low, that solves the problem of obesity, meaning you will be thin for the rest of your life, your blood pressure will be ok, tiredness after meals will be finished and there is less inflammation, which means less Alzheimer's, heart attacks, strokes, cancers, and depression to name just a few.

Now you want to know how to keep your insulin low. If I tell you what to do, will you say, "It is too difficult to stop eating the things I like the most?" See it as a smoker who is intoxicated by cigarettes and wants to stop. But, when he does stop, he will have withdrawal symptoms.

To succeed in your new life, (the former was high insulin, the new life is low insulin), you have to overcome the withdrawal symptoms that will last about one week. These symptoms will be low energy, fatigue, and depression.

What I am about to tell you will change your life, but only if you take it seriously and decide to pilot your body, which is a sophisticated machine that needs a good driver (a good pilot). Until now, you have been putting a lot of things in your mouth that are not food. If it tastes good, it does not automatically mean it is good for your body. A lot of time is spent by your body fighting the things (not good food) that you did put in your mouth. No wonder people become tired, depressed, and overweight. For the rest of your life, you are going to make a decision before you put anything in your mouth.

The decision will be "yes" or "no." Is that food for humans or some stuff that can be eaten? It may taste good, but is not good food for humans. To check if you are still with us, the bad food (not human food) increases insulin, creates inflammation, and makes you sick. Good human food keeps insulin low, makes you feel good, productive, and happy to be.

Now some history on what is human food.

Our genes are 40,000 years old and for the first

30,000 years, humans were eating the hunter-gatherer diet or what is called today the Paleolithic diet—meat, fish, poultry, eggs, vegetables, fruits, nuts, and olive oil. The principle is simple. If you stay on that diet and there are no restrictions on quantity, your insulin will stay low, obesity and diabetes will be gone, high blood pressure gets better, and tiredness after meals is gone.

In the last 10,000 years, the agricultural era, new items to eat became accessible to humans. Most of them (flour, cereals, rice, potatoes, and sweet liquids) increase insulin production by the pancreas because they are quickly absorbed glucides (carbohydrates). This means they do not remain in the intestine a long time and sugar will increase in the blood shortly after eating.

This high sugar in the blood after meals provokes a lot of insulin secretion in order to park that sugar outside of the blood vessels, toward the liver and the fat cells. So, you get fat and have a liver that is called fatty liver. These new foods also include cereals, flour, pasta, rice, potatoes, sugar, and milk.

What you eat has more importance than you think on the way you feel! But all this description of food has to be put in context. Humans do not react equally toward food. Some can eat cereals, pasta, rice, potatoes, and they do not gain weight, their insulin stays low and they feel good. Even some of those people feel bad when they eat meat. They have adapted to the new food from the agricultural era.

But, for the ones who gain weight easily when they

eat cereals, pasta, rice, potatoes, and sugar, they should know we are adapted to the Paleolithic era and should eat only meat, fish, poultry, eggs, vegetables, fruits, and nuts. The goal is to keep our level of insulin low.

This way, I believe (I know), that every day you are going to feel better and the degenerative diseases such as diabetes, obesity, and all other problems that are caused by high sugar and high insulin, will be avoided.

Could it be that simple? The answer is YES!

The decision is yours! Can you stop eating the things you like the most?

You know all the smokers who stopped are happy they did, even if in the first two or three months they were not sure. After a while you will discover a new taste and you will never want to go back to the food (the quickly absorbed glucides) that were making you sick, not energetic and may I say, obese. I am a little hard on you because I gave you the explanation and the recipe to feeling good, energetic and physically fit! Can you do it?

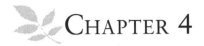

CHAPTER 4

Medications, Drugs, Supplements, Pills and Hormones

These terms need to be defined so that you and I understand the same thing. Because I would like to help you in the decisions you make regarding pills.

If I succeed, your choice of taking a pill will be based more on facts than faith.

Some things are necessary for our bodies, vitamin C for example. We do not make it, but we need to take it as a supplement in fruits or pills so our body will not be deficient.

Another thing that belongs in the body is the thyroid hormone. We do make it but if our production is not enough, we will have a deficiency. Symptoms such as fatigue and weight gain will appear. The treatment is to take a thyroid hormone supplement.

Think of it as oil in your car. You check the oil and if it is low, you add the right quantity so the oil level will be perfect. The point here is that the oil belongs in your car. There can be no side effect from adjusting the oil level to perfection. This is the same thing for all the hormones that belong in your body—to adjust them to perfect (optimum) levels. This cannot have a bad effect. It will only reestablish the optimal function of that hormone.

Some things do not belong to the body—aspirin for example. We do not make it and the body does not need it to function properly. And it does not exist in nature, even if it is made from a natural product (salicylic acid). If you have a headache, the cause of the headache is not a lack of aspirin in your system. When you take an aspirin for a headache, you do not treat the cause, you only reduce the levels of cytokine that were high. The headache may go away, but there are always side effects when you use medications or drugs that do not belong to the body. When deciding whether to take a drug or medication, you have to figure the plus and the minus.

In the short term, in emergency situations, the drugs or medication have good results, but, for chronic problems, it is better to look for the cause of the problem.

Some things do not belong to the body, such as natural products. We do not make them and the body does not need them to function properly. But, they do exist in nature, which means we can use them without a doctor's prescription. They are used to alter the body's physiology to our advantage, meaning more plus than minus. Most natural products are safe—meaning, they rarely kill.

Remember, even if natural products exist in nature, our body does not need them to function properly. They do not treat the cause and they have side effects. They should be used like drugs or medications, with good knowledge of the advantages and the side effects.

I divided the pills into four categories:

1. Things that are part of the body that the body needs to function properly, but we do not produce by ourselves. They are vitamins (A, B, C, D, and E), minerals (iodine, selenium, zinc, etc.), and oils (omega-3, 6, and 9). We need to eat them or take them as a supplement. Note: Do not take supplements of omega-6 because the American diet already contains too much.

2. Things that belong to the body that the body needs to function properly, but we do produce by ourselves. They are the hormones (thyroid, melatonin, estrogen, testosterone, progesterone, DHEA, cortisone and growth hormone, etc.), and there are enzymes or co-enzymes (CoQ10, alpha lipoic acid, acetyl-L-carnitine, etc.). The hormones need to be monitored, like the oil in your car, and supplemented if not at an ideal level. The enzymes and coenzymes can

be taken as a supplement, because aging reduces their production.

3. Things that are not part of the body, which the body does not need to function properly, and that do not exist in nature. They are the drugs, the medications created by humans (antibiotics, blood pressure pills, diabetes pill, etc.). This industry is highly regulated and the proof of efficiency is well documented. They require prescriptions and should be monitored for side effects.

4. Things that do not belong to the body, that the body does not need to function properly, that do exist in nature. They are the natural products (curcumin, saw palmetto, resveratrol, etc.) They are usually safe. They can have side effects, but they can be beneficial if used judiciously.

Where do we go now? Before adding a new molecule into your body, first try to check if the ones that belong to your body are there and in the ideal quantity. I want you to understand that if you want to be well and healthy, you first have to take care of category one and two. Eat well and take the supplements (vitamins, minerals, and hormones) to be sure that all the needs of your body are satisfied. Find a doctor who can test and question you about your hormones, to be sure they are at their optimum levels. Adjust what should be in your body at optimum levels: vitamins; minerals; hormones; and enzymes.

Second, stop bad behavior that intoxicated you, such as eating food that is bad for you, including sugar, using alcohol or tobacco, and living a bad lifestyle.

Third, use medications or drugs (synonymous for me) for a short term, to help the symptoms while you look for the cause of the problem.

Note: Iron should not be part of a multivitamin. Iron should be supplemented only in people proved to be deficient by a blood test. People who take an "iron supplement" when they do not need it, will have a shorter life. More on that later in the iron chapter.

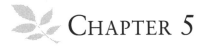

CHAPTER 5

Sugar

"Sugar" is something that you should use as a swear word—it is not something that you should eat. Before the agricultural era, you could not find sugar in a pure concentrated form. It was mostly mixed with fibers in fruits. Meaning, when you eat fruit, the fibers slow the absorption of the sugar, which stays longer in the intestines before it goes to the bloodstream. That is good because there is less spike of sugar in the blood.

But when you eat the pure sugar you get from sweet liquids, desserts, flour, pasta, rice, and potatoes, you will have a spike of sugar in the blood that you will have to fight. What kind of fight? When you have type 2 diabetes, it means you lost the fight against sugar! Sugar is always high and insulin is always high. Both sugar and insulin contribute to the damage and inflammation that destroys your body at a high speed.

When you eat sugar and you are not diabetic yet, your body secretes insulin to lower the sugar in the blood. With success, you think? Then think twice. Where does that sugar go? It goes to the liver! When the liver is full, it becomes what we call fatty liver—a pre-cirrhosis condition. It goes into the fat cells, meaning you get bigger and those fat cells secrete inflammatory cytokines, which make you sick. So by eating sugar you start a war in your body that you cannot win.

Where else can that sugar go? The more sugar you eat, the more it will have to find a place to be stored as triglycerides, fat, or as glycogen in the liver.

Our endothelium are the cells lining the inside of our blood vessels. These cells are very active when healthy. They secrete nitric oxide which, in the right quantity, keeps our blood vessels open. This means good blood pressure, good circulation in general, and good erectile function. I think you get the picture!

When you eat sugar, it goes into your endothelium cells and will make them sick. Those endothelium cells will secrete less nitric oxide and the first sign of this will be higher blood pressure.

Now you can figure out the rest. When those endothelium cells are sick, they will not repair themselves as well. High sugar and high insulin contribute to the inflammation in the inside lining of the blood vessels (endothelium) and that inflammation will create acne on the face and a similar reaction in the blood vessels. This will build plaque and lead to obstruction of the blood circulation. If this happens in the blood vessels that feed the heart's coronary artery, it can cause a heart attack. If it happens in a blood vessel that feeds the brain, it is a stroke. It can happen in any blood vessel.

When you eat sugar, you lose a battle and it takes around 20 years to lose the war. Meaning, when a blood vessel gets so damaged that an obstruction occurs, you get a heart attack or stroke.

An important point to understand is when your body is fighting sugar, you lose a lot of energy that you cannot use to perform at your optimum because insulin will transport the sugar inside every cell of your body. All those cells have a function—work to do. That function will be reduced by the intoxication of too much sugar!

I said that it takes around 20 years of high insulin levels before the blood vessels suffer enough damage for an obstruction to happen. Earlier generations started to eat more sugar, bread, pasta, rice, and potatoes only later in their life, after the 1970s when everybody started the war on fat. They were having their heart attacks after 55 years of age. Now, the new generation was raised with a low-fat diet; meaning more sugar. They are obese earlier in life and are having heart attacks at a younger age.

Now, I did talk about heart attacks without saying cholesterol because it is not the cholesterol that causes heart attacks. It is the chronic inflammation that is caused by the oxidation (a rust-like reaction) of a protein that carries the cholesterol or the LDL (low density lipoprotein) that contributes to the formation of plaque in the blood vessels. This means that if cholesterol is there and there is no inflammation, the blood vessels will be healthy.

Low-density lipoprotein carries the cholesterol to the site of use. Like a postman delivers the post. We need it. It has an important function—to deliver cholesterol where it is needed. When we eat too much sugar, those LDLs have a tendency to become smaller and oxidized. They get trapped in the inflammation of the blood vessels and will contribute to the formation of plaque (a bad scar inside of blood vessels).

Inflammation is caused by a high-sugar diet, yes. But other causes of inflammation are low vitamin D, trans fat, food allergies (milk, eggs, gluten and others), intolerance, bad intestinal flora, hormonal imbalances, high homocysteine, toxins (xenobiotic, pesticides, heavy metals, etc.), and chronic infection (helicobacter pylori in the stomach, gingivitis in the gums).

A word on high-fructose corn syrup. The sugar that is produced from corn syrup is chemically transformed to have a higher fructose ratio because it is sweeter and less is then needed for a sweet taste. This kind of sugar creates bigger spikes of insulin, meaning the body reacts strongly to high fructose corn syrup; meaning more insulin equals more inflammation. It will make you diabetic faster. That is the sugar most commonly used in the soft drink industry.

If you decide to reduce or stop your sugar intake, be aware that your body is adapted to fighting the sugar by producing high amounts of insulin. So, for the first week of stopping sugar consumption, your insulin will still be higher than it needs to be and you will feel bad sugar cravings and tiredness. It can be difficult. But after one week, I do promise you will feel great and the withdrawal symptoms will stop!

Can sugar be eaten? Yes. It is while you exercise heavily and in the one hour after exercising. The reason is that if sugar is taken during exercise, it will not make insulin secretions, because insulin is secreted only after blood sugar increases. While exercising, if you drink or eat sugar (not too much), the blood sugar will not increase because the working cells aspirate sugar from the blood.

So the next time you drop something or bad things happen to you, swear instead by saying "SUGAR!" and you will preach that sugar is bad.

CHAPTER 6

Cholesterol

Cholesterol is a fatty molecule, meaning it is soluble in fat, not in water. The blood is a water-like solution. That means that cholesterol needs a protein to bind to, in order to be transported in the blood. Those proteins are LDL (low density lipoprotein) and HDL (high density lipoprotein).

Cholesterol is mostly made by the liver. If you eat more cholesterol, your liver will make less, adjusting itself to the need. If you eat less cholesterol, your liver will make more, adjusting to the need. The need? Yes—cholesterol is needed!

Cholesterol has the building blocks for the body's steroid hormones, such as cortisone, DHEA, testosterone, estrogen, progesterone, androstenedione, pregnenolone, and vitamin D. Steroid means made from "chole-sterol." These hormones are very important for the proper functioning of the body.

Steroid hormones are produced in many places in the

body such as testicles, ovaries, and adrenals. These glands work hard to produce the steroid hormones we need. With age and toxic contamination, their production is reduced and, when that happens, the brain and the body receive less of these precious steroid hormones, and a mechanism tells the liver to increase the production of CHOLESTEROL.

So low steroid hormone, caused by aging, toxicity, or an inborn error of metabolism, is the reason for high cholesterol. The associated increase in diseases, seen when cholesterol is high, is mostly caused by the low steroid hormones, not by cholesterol itself. Fifty percent of people who have a heart attack (blockage of a coronary artery) have a normal level of cholesterol.

When the liver increases its production of cholesterol, the body is trying to repair itself by making more of the building blocks (cholesterol) to produce more steroid hormones. But this does not work because the glands that make the steroid hormones are damaged. So the cholesterol will stay high until you take supplements of the steroid hormones that are low. The cholesterol will go back to normal if you take supplements to adjust your steroid hormones to optimum levels.

Note: Thyroid hormone supplements lower the cholesterol too, but by a different mechanism. Thyroid hormones stimulate the excretion of cholesterol in the bile so, when thyroid hormones are low, less cholesterol is excreted in the bile (i.e. into the intestine then outside of the body).

Is cholesterol bad? Cholesterol is a crucial molecule in your body. Steroid hormones are made from it. Also, cholesterol is a very important material in the membranes of every cell of your body. Cell membranes should be made of cholesterol, DHA and EPA (omega-3), gamma linoleic ac (omega-6) and omega-9. These fats are called essential fatty acids. Cell membranes should not be made of trans fat.

Here you see the importance of eating well. When trans fat gets into the making of the membranes of your brain cells, heart cells, etc., these membranes become more rigid than normal. Trans fat is a toxic material that should not come into the making of your cell membranes because those cells will not function well.

Any oil can become trans fat if heated enough by high temperature cooking, such as grilling or frying. Some oils are better at resisting the heat before they become trans fat, such as coconut oil and butter. So, think twice before eating fried food. The damage will last for months. And think twice before letting your kids eat fried food. The damage will last for years.

What is the good cholesterol? It is HDL (high-density lipoprotein), a protein that takes the cholesterol from all over the body where it has not been used and carries it back to the liver for processing and evacuation in the bile. It is called the good cholesterol, but it is a protein. It is not cholesterol, since its function is to make a cleaning of cholesterol. Everybody agrees that it is good. People who have a high HDL are healthier, have fewer heart attacks, and mainly in women, it protects their blood vessels from inflammation and obstruction.

You can increase your HDL by eating animal fat (organically raised) cooked at low temperatures or boiled, and by exercising.

The bad reputation of animal fat comes when it is cooked at high temperatures (grilled or fried). It becomes trans fat and/or A.G.E. (Advance Glycation End Product), a toxic product of cooking, and this fat transformation from the chemical reaction that occurs when cooked at high temperatures is to blame. So it is the cooking of animal fat at high temperatures that creates the unwanted inflammation. Animal fat cooked at low temperatures, such as in a crock pot, is better because it increases the HDL or the good cholesterol protein.

What is the bad cholesterol? It is LDL (low density lipoprotein). This is a protein that carries the cholesterol from the liver, where it is made, to the sites where it is needed; to the glands that make steroid hormones; to the brain; and to all the cells of your body or their membrane construction. So far this sounds good, but the problem with LDL is that the proteins come in different sizes. The smaller they get, the more they are sensitive to oxidation (like rust on your car).

When the LDL are oxidized, they will get involved in the inflammation occurring in your blood vessels and make it worse, meaning more bad plaques in blood vessels. Oxidation of LDL happens when triglycerides are high, when HDL is low, and when insulin is high.

The solution is to keep the size of LDL big by eating animal fat (organic) cooked at low temperatures; keep triglycerides low by eating less or no sugar, bread, flour, rice and pasta; and keep insulin low by not eating sugar, bread, flour, rice, pasta, desserts, and sweet liquids.

To keep the LDL quantity low is good. Keep triglycerides and insulin low by not eating sugar, bread, flour, pasta, rice and potatoes. It is mostly the sugar and fast-absorbed glucides that are bad for the blood vessels. The fat that is bad is the trans fat.

If you want to reduce your cholesterol and LDL and increase HDL, you must reduce or stop eating sugar, bread, flour, pasta, rice, potatoes, and trans fat. You can increase animal fat by cooking only organically grown meat at low temperatures and increasing your exercise. By doing that, if your blood pressure was high, it will get to normal. And your risk of heart attack and stroke will be lowered significantly. Your risk of cancer will be reduced too.

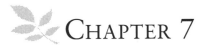

CHAPTER 7

Diabetes (Type 2)

What an ugly name. It has the advantage of no one wanting to be a diabetic. Is there diabetes (type 2), high blood pressure, or obesity in your family? Some say that you are genetically predisposed to become a diabetic. So what do you want to do?

Eat what the other diabetics (type 2) eat and become like them because you like the taste of those foods. And when you try to stop eating sugar, cereal, flour, bread, pasta, rice, potatoes, and sweet liquids, you have sugar cravings. So you think you need sugar and quickly absorbed carbohydrates. Or can you listen to what I have to say and understand it?

Usually diabetes is a condition that makes you feel bad most of the time. Diabetics (type 2) have a tendency to feel better when they eat (good or bad food). When a diabetic eats bad food, he might have 30 minutes of satisfaction and 24 hours of suffering. That is the reason why diabetics have a tendency to eat frequently.

The goal of my intervention today is to convince you to eat good food and still have the satisfaction after eating, but not the suffering that comes later. When you eat bad food, it makes spikes of insulin secretion and you have the side effects of high insulin. So the secret is to keep insulin low.

What happens inside diabetics with type 2 is, when they eat sugar in any form (sweet liquids, cereal, bread, flour, pasta, rice, potatoes, desserts, etc.), that sugar quickly enters the bloodstream from the intestine. Then the reaction of the body is to secrete insulin from the pancreas to send away that sugar to a parking area that is inside the liver (which leads to fatty liver), into the fat cells (leading to obesity), and into all the cells of your body until they are full.

When all the body is full, we call it insulin resistance. That means that even when the insulin level is very high in the blood, it does not succeed in lowering the blood sugar. If you are a diabetic, you are full of inflammation because your body is trying to fight what you put in your mouth, which is destroying the optimum physiology that your body needs.

The inflammation caused by high sugar and high insulin makes you feel sick and tired (mostly after meals), increases cancer and diseases of any kind from infections to heart attacks and strokes. Do I need to say more?

I told you earlier that often diabetics do not listen to good advice. This is because they feel better when they eat and the advice given to them is to stop eating the things they like. So they are afraid to feel bad all the time.

The solution to the dilemma is in insulin physiology. Insulin is a hormone that we have to keep low in order to optimize the necessary functions of the body. When insulin is high, its effects may last four to six hours. But often the sugar will be lowered earlier. This means low blood sugar will happen, which results in feeling shaky and craving sugar.

For the first week, when you adopt a diet that keeps insulin low, your pancreas will still make too much insulin because it was trained to adapt to the former diet of eating sugar. This means, for the first week of not eating sweet liquids, bread, flour, pasta, rice, or potatoes, you will not feel well and you will have the symptoms of too high insulin, such as tiredness and sugar craving. But after around one week of not cheating, you will experience the new you!

This means feeling better, experiencing weight loss without eating fewer calories and, in weeks to a month, you will no longer be a diabetic and experience lower blood pressure. The cause of diabetes is the food ingested! The cure for diabetes (type 2) is not to eat the food that causes diabetes.

If you want to become diabetic, you should eat sweet liquids, cereal, flour, bread, pasta, rice, potatoes, and sweets in quantities that will make your blood sugar increase and your insulin levels increase.

If you want to avoid diabetes, obesity, and high blood pressure, you should reduce eating what causes diabetes. By eating less or none at all of the quickly absorbed glucides (carbohydrates), you are going to eat more of the slowly absorbed glucides, which include vegetables and fruits.

You should also increase the good fats. These include animal fat (organic, cooked at low temperatures), omega-3 (fish oil), omega-9 (olive oil, avocados), and nuts such as peanuts, almonds, macadamias, and cashews.

You see diabetes has a cause and if you avoid the cause, there is no more diabetes! Could it be that simple? YES! It works all the time.

In summary, if you are a diabetic (type 2) or your chances of becoming one is high, you should adopt a diet that is called the Paleolithic diet from the era before agriculture.

You should not eat:

Bread, cereal, flour, pasta, rice, potatoes
Sweet liquids (not even orange juice)
Desserts, dried fruits
Dairy products (check chapter on dairy)

You should eat:

Meat, fish, eggs, poultry (organic, cooked at
low temperatures)
Vegetables and legumes (very diversified)
Fruits (fresh, not dried)
Nuts (peanuts, almonds, etc.)
Olive oil and lemon juice (for salad dressing)
Butter or coconut oil for cooking (because they
tolerate the heat better, before becoming
trans fat). When the butter changes
to a brown color while cooking, it has
become trans fat and it is too late.

Now you know the facts—the ball is in your court.

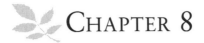 CHAPTER 8

High Blood Pressure Hypertension

This disease can kill you, but it takes time. You don't experience many symptoms, so you don't seek treatment unless you are fearful that hypertension is a risk factor for coronary heart disease, stroke, renal failure, or peripheral vascular disease (blockage of the leg artery).

Five to ten percent of hypertension patients have a secondary cause, such as chronic renal disease, hypothyroidism, or hyperthyroidism. For the other 90%, the cause is what you eat that keeps insulin high, leading to inflammation in your blood vessels. That inflammation restrains the endothelium (the inside thin cell layer of your blood vessels) from making enough nitric oxide and not enough nitric oxide can lead to hypertension. If we understand how blood pressure is maintained normally, we will understand why it becomes too high.

Normal blood pressure is 120/80. This means 120 at the peak when the heart contracts and 80 at the lowest just before the heart contracts again.

High blood pressure is diagnosed when the first number is higher than 140 and/or the second number is higher than 90.

Blood pressure has to be taken with precision. You should be sitting for at least 15 minutes with your arm at rest. Some patients have what we call "white-coat hypertension." This means they have high readings only when somebody takes their blood pressure. When an automatic machine takes the blood pressure during 24 hours, their readings are normal. This is because of the anxiety of having blood pressure taken by medical personnel.

Blood pressure varies all the time—when you stand, you move, it's cold, it's hot, etc. This is for a good reason. It is the pressure of the blood that makes the blood flow to all the organs of our body—brain, muscles, kidneys, etc. So our blood pressure is maintained by a very fancy system so each organ will have the right amount of blood it needs in different situations.

The heart pumps the blood through vessels that are like pipes. But the blood vessels are not like rigid copper pipes that you have in your house. Blood vessels are elastic. They have a muscle layer that can vary their caliber or their diameter. The important point is that by default, they have a tendency to constrict and reduce their diameter. This offers resistance to blood flow, which causes high blood pressure. If by default, all our blood vessels have a tendency to constrict, by what mechanism can we maintain a normal blood pressure?

This mechanism is the endothelium, the inner lining of our blood vessels, which, when healthy, secretes a substance called nitric oxide. That nitric oxide is secreted into the blood flow and lasts 10 seconds. It does its job— being absorbed in the blood vessel's flesh. This releases the tension in the muscles of the blood vessel. The blood vessels become bigger in size (diameter), the blood flow increases and blood pressure becomes normal.

So high blood pressure happens when our endothelium is sick and does not produce enough nitric oxide.

Mechanisms that cause our endothelium to get sick include:

Eating an inflammatory diet: high sugar and quickly
      absorbed glucides (high insulin)

Too much alcohol

Too much caffeine

Too much stress

Not enough exercise

Not enough essential fatty acid, omega-3

Not enough vitamin D

Heavy metal toxins: lead and cadmium are known to
cause hypertension

Dairy products (in some sensitive patients).

Now that you understand how your blood pressure

gets high, maybe I have a chance to convince you to change your lifestyle because it is the lifestyle that causes most of the cases of hypertension. High blood pressure was rarely seen in former civilizations.

Some people eat like other people, but they do not suffer from hypertension. This is because they are less sensitive than you are. If you have hypertension and you decide to change your lifestyle, you are going to cure not just your blood pressure, but all the other conditions that are caused by a poor lifestyle, such as fatigue (mostly after meals), being overweight, suffering chronic articular pain, frequent headaches, etc.

First adopt the Paleolithic diet. This will lower your insulin, inflammation, weight, etc.

You should eat:

Meat, fish, eggs, poultry (all organic, cooked at low
    temperatures)
Vegetables, legumes (beans)
Fruits (fresh, not dried)
Nuts
Olive oil (for dressing)
Butter or coconut oil (for cooking)

Do not eat:

Flour, cereal, bread, pasta, rice, potatoes
Sweet liquid (not even juice of any kind)
Sweets of any kind: dessert; candy; dried fruit; etc.
Dairy products (for sensitive patients)

Stop for one month and you will see the difference. I also recommend taking some supplements (your doctor should agree):

Recommended Supplements:

Vitamin D – 2000-5000 international units per day

Vitamin C – 1000 mg twice per day

Magnesium – (if you do not have renal insufficiency problems) 500 mg per day.

Fish oil – EPA 1000 mg, DHA 500 mg per day

Be sure that your thyroid function is considered optimum and, if you take a multivitamin plus minerals, make sure that it does not contain iron. Iron supplements for someone not deficient in iron can shorten their lifespan.

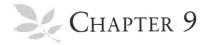

CHAPTER 9

What To Eat

What you should eat depends on who you are! Cats should eat cat food. If they eat food that is not for them, they will be sick, with fur problems, behavior problems, and so on. Humans are omnivores, which means they CAN eat very diversified types of food. But it does not mean that they SHOULD eat everything. The human race is very diversified. Some people can eat cereals, flour, and grain products, but others cannot because they have gluten intolerance. People who are very active can eat some sugar, but the sedentary person should not eat sugar.

Humans are the only animals that eat dairy (milk, cheese, yogurt) after they are weaned. Think about it. If you are healthy with no problems, you can continue to eat dairy products. But if you are feeling sick and have symptoms such as feeling tired, or suffering from breast tenderness, bloating, high blood pressure, easy weight gain, or migraines, you should try stopping dairy products for one month. If you feel better, this means dairy was not for you. If you see no difference, then you may resume eating dairy.

Some people feel good when they eat cereals, such as flour, bread, pasta, rice, or potatoes. They have a tendency to be vegetarians. When they eat meat, they feel bad. They are adapted to the agricultural era and also have a tendency to be blood type A.

Some people feel good when they eat meat. They are adapted to the Paleolithic era. The meat eater has a tendency to be blood type 0. Those adapted to the Paleolithic era have a tendency to feel bad when they cereals, flour, sugar, and dairy because they secrete high amounts of insulin anytime sugar gets into their system.

That insulin secreted in high amounts creates a yo-yo effect of blood sugar. This means, after they eat sugar, insulin gets high, then sugar gets too low, then they crave sugar again. You get the picture. Those humans should not eat sugar, cereals, or flour products (bread, pasta), rice, or potatoes. And it is obvious—no sweet liquids.

In some studies, red meat has a bad reputation. Red meat can be toxic if cooked at high temperatures, like over charcoal in a barbecue. It is the black, overcooked part that is not good for you.

But if you cook your red meat in a slow cooker or crock pot or use any low-temperature cooking technique, then red meat is all right to eat.

Cattle should eat beef food. That is grass and hay. Grass and hay contain omega-3. When cattle eat it, their meat will contain omega-3. But now cattle are fed with grains, which grow faster, but their meat no longer contains any omega-3. Also, the pesticides used for pest control in farming works their way into the beef meat. So when you eat farm animals, choose organically raised. It is not without poison, but contains less.

Prepared foods are designed to taste good and have a long shelf life.

Therefore, they may contain additives, like nitrates, salt, and MSG (monosodium glutamate). They are second-quality foods. You must read the labels. You have to learn to read a label and when the label is too long, I would not eat it.

High-fructose corn syrup is a sugar made from corn instead of sugar cane. High-fructose corn syrup contains 30% more fructose than sugar cane and tastes more sweet. But it also creates more insulin secretion when you drink it. So it will make you a diabetic faster. Sweet liquids are not recommended except for those who are very active. But the high fructose from corn syrup should be avoided by all. Most of the sweetener in the pop/soda industry is high fructose from corn syrup.

Some sweeteners with no calories are made from foreign molecules that are from new, space-age technology. Will our bodies be able to adapt to it? Do you want to be part of the experiment? Some are from a plant called stevia, which means it is natural. Can our bodies adapt to a large amount of a natural product. This is an experiment too!

One product called Xylitol is said to protect against dental cavities. But why are there dental cavities in the first place? The cause is bad bacteria (streptococcus mutans) that grow in your mouth when you eat sugar. Your saliva can clean your mouth in 15 minutes after you eat sugar. So, if you drink a sweet liquid and sip every fifteen minutes, that's the route to more dental cavities. If you are prone to dental cavities, Xylitol gum may help you. But do not forget that this is an experiment and we do not know the long-term side effects.

All in all, when you consume an artificial sweetener, you LIE to your body. Your taste buds will think that sugar is coming and a message is sent to the pancreas to prepare insulin for the sugar coming. But none will come. This insulin that was prepared may be released into the blood stream, then low blood sugar will happen and you will crave sugar. Eat sugar, feel better, and gain weight. The reason you were eating artificial sweetener in the beginning (not to gain weight) is lost.

One study showed that people who drink one diet soda per day gained more weight than people who drink one regular soda per day. This was a one-month study. The explanation is, when you consume artificial sweeteners, you have a tendency to eat more of other sugar. My recommendation is do yourself a favor and stop lying to your body. Do not use those things that taste sweet but are a lie.

Nutrition is a passion for many—sometimes it can be like a religion.

The goal of eating is to feed our body the things that it needs to function at optimum levels. The best foods are the fresh ones with less possible toxic chemicals in them. For example, a juice is a transformed product, while the best food is fresh fruit. In a grocery store, the fresh foods are around the store. The alleys in between are where the transformed products are sold.

Chocolate is a transformed product that contains cacao (percentage listed on label) and sugar. Cacao is good. Sugar is not good. A good compromise is to eat a little quantity of 85% cacao, with 15% sugar. That's a good deal!

In 1970s, fat was blamed for all the heart attacks. At that time, a lot of fat consumed was in the form of trans fat and all fats were treated equally. Even now! All fats are not equal. Some are very, very good, some are good, and trans fat is bad.

Some fats are called essential fatty acids and they are very good. These include omega-3 (fish oil), omega-6 (linoleic acid, gamma linoleic acids), omega-9 (nuts, olive oil, avocado).

Animal fat is good when cooked at low temperatures. Animal fat is good because it improves the lipid profile (increases HDL, increases the size of the LDL, reduces the triglycerides). It also lowers insulin (which is good).

The effect of a higher fat diet (50% of total calories) means lower inflammation, less sugar swings (up and down), a thinner body, and no sugar craving.

So try to figure out who you are in the human race. Then decide what kind of food you can eat and you should eat for optimum performance. An example to help you is if you have a tendency to gain weight easily, the foods that you should avoid are: sweet liquids; bread; flour; pasta; rice; potatoes; sweets; and desserts—all the things that you like a lot. But that's it. Do it and the problem is solved.

I don't want to be hard on you, but this is because of high insulin secretion when you add sugar and low activity, which can lead to obesity. You should eat the Paleolithic diet (fish, eggs, poultry, vegetables, fruit, nuts, and olive oil).

I will have more in the chapter on obesity.

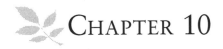

CHAPTER 10

Kids' Menus

Children's menus in restaurants are usually junk food – mostly fried things that I do not considered food. Who is responsible for giving food to the children?

Should the children decide what they should eat themselves? Should we call youth protection when kids eat at restaurants?

Because the food we eat is what makes our body structure, growing children are more sensitive to the intake of nutrients, proteins (amino acids), good fats, bad fats, good carbohydrates and bad carbohydrates, for the making of brains, bones, muscles, nerves, etc. All parents act as examples to their children. Should they eat in front of their children? Am I trying to make trouble here or am I sounding the alarm?

Let me tell you a true story. One day at my office, I saw a diabetic lady for a follow-up visit. As usual, I taught good nutrition—avoidance of all the quickly absorbed glucides (no sweet liquids, no pasta, no bread, etc.). That evening, I went to a convenience store and who do I see coming out the door but that diabetic patient with 24 cans of orange soda in her arms. She stared at me with anxiety and told me it was not what I thought—it was for the kids! So the kids are not diabetic yet from drinking sodas, but they will get a chance to become diabetic at an early age. Is that what the mother wants? No, but it is what she does!

So I think that some parents are unaware of the consequences of bad eating habits. The most common excuse is the "only sometimes" defense, but to me "sometimes" seems quite often. Most chronic diseases and inflammation are caused by bad food, lack of essential nutrients, fatty acids, amino acids, vitamins, minerals, and too much sugar. Most bad fats are the ones transformed by cooking at high temperatures. Most bad sugars are the ones that are quickly absorbed from the gut into the blood.

Children like the taste of sugar, but that does not mean it is good for them. Sugar is not good for children. Sugar is not good for anybody. Fried (in oil) food is not good for the young, nor the grown-up.

What is good then for the children? The same thing that is good for all humans:

• Fish, meat, eggs, poultry—cooked at low temperatures and yes, animal fat is good if cooked at low temperatures in a crock pot or boiled.

• Vegetables—all kinds, moderately cooked;

- Beans;
- Good oils—omega-3 from fish, omega-9 from olive oil or avocados;
- Nuts—peanuts, cashews, almonds, etc., cooked at low temperatures;
- Fruits—up to five per day. They are the desserts;
- Water (all sweet liquids are to be avoided, including orange juice).

Salt is ok. Sugar is not ok! So what should be avoided and what should be reduced?

In the avoidance category are:

Everything that is fried at high temperatures (French fries, nuggets, fried chicken, potatoes, chips, etc.).

Sweet liquids (all sodas and even all fruit juices).

In the reduce category are:

All flours, bread, pasta, cereals, etc.

All desserts (eat fruits instead).

Dairy products (milk is a sweet liquid and contain casein, a protein that is difficult to digest). Yogurt is also a sweet liquid.

The next question is should children take vitamin supplements? The answer lies in what our children are most deficient in. The answer is the deficiency in vitamins and minerals varies depending on what you eat and where you live. They are mostly vitamin D, vitamin A and vitamin C. I recommend giving a supplement of vitamins to all children. By giving a safe dosage, I think that everyone will benefit without adverse effects.

The dosage is:

From 0 to 2 years old: vitamin A, 1500 international units per day; vitamin C, 30 mg per day; vitamin D, 400 international units per day.

From 2 to 12 years old: roughly double the dosage.

After 12 years of age, you can give the adult dosage. That is: vitamin A, 10,000 iu/day; vitamin C, 500-1000 mg twice per day; and vitamin D, 2000-5000 iu/day.

Good nutrition does not seem to happen by luck. Somebody has to take charge and the parents are in the best position!

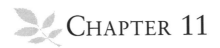

CHAPTER 11

Cooking of Food

(The Missing Link in Nutrition)

We cook food to be sure it's dead with no microorganism attached to it. But cooking is a chemistry game that we play whether we like chemistry or not.

Have you heard of the Maillard Reaction, AGE (Advanced Glycation End Product), acrylamide, lipid peroxide, or cholesterol oxide? They are the very toxic products that are produced by cooking food at high temperatures (higher than 240 F or 120 C). The best way to cook food is by boiling or steaming at temperatures lower than 240 F or 120 C, in a crock pot, for example.

When food (protein, amino acids, sugar and lipids) is cooked at high temperatures, its chemical structure is changed. What you start with is not what ends up on your plate after it is cooked.

The two most known toxins produced by cooking

are Advanced Glycation End Products, also called glycotoxins, and acrylamide.

AGE (Advanced Glycation End Products) are very toxic when eaten. They cause an increase of C-reactive protein and an increase of TNF-alpha, two bad things that provoke premature aging and increased inflammation. These are highly related to cardiovascular diseases, allergies, diabetes, Alzheimer's, rheumatoid arthritis, osteoarthritis, kidney diseases, and cancer. Specific receptors for AGE have recently been identified and their toxicity recognized. This is why most doctors and nutritionists do not know yet the worst effects of those toxins on human physiology.

Acrylamide is an AGE or a glycotoxine. It is toxic to the neurons (nervous system) and also is a known carcinogen (provokes cancer). It is made from the amino acid asparagine, which is in starch (potatoes, cereals). You find acrylamide mainly in cookies, French fries, and potato chips.

You do not want AGE and acrylamide in your body. They are difficult to avoid and the best way to reduce the quantity you eat is to cook at low temperatures. Steaming is the very best method because you lose fewer nutrients. Boiling is second best.

But it is not good to fry food! But fried food will still exist. When fried, food becomes toxic in two ways. AGE (Advance Glycation End Product) is created and also the oil you use is transformed into oxidized fat and trans fat (toxic). So I advise using oil that is more heat stable, such as coconut oil, peanut oil, or olive oil.

Some vitamins are also heat sensitive, meaning they are destroyed by cooking. They are vitamin C, vitamin B1 (thiamine), folate (the real vitamin B9), and vitamin B12. Iodine added to the salt is also volatile. If you add iodized salt to the food before it is cooked, then, during cooking, the iodine will evaporate into the air.

Microwave cooking is a kind of high temperature cooking (not good). When you use aluminum cookware, aluminum is leaching into the food while cooking (not good) and aluminum intoxication is known to increase osteoporosis and Alzheimer's.

We store food in airtight containers in a refrigerator to prevent cholesterol from oxidizing (toxic for blood vessels) and to prevent polyunsaturated fatty acids from oxidizing into toxic lipid peroxides, etc. For storing foods, containers made of glass are better than those made of plastic. Plastics contain phthalate and biphenyl, which are endocrine disruptors that leach from the plastic, get into the food and then into you. Phthalate and biphenyl from plastics are possible contributors to diabetes, cancer, sperm abnormalities, miscarriage, premature breast development, and autoimmune disease.

The food you eat can be altered by cooking and by the storage. The recommendations in this chapter are very important for a healthy lifestyle.

CHAPTER 12

Food Allergy

According to one estimate, as much as 60% of people suffer from undetected food allergies. Reported symptoms vary quite a bit and often are outside of the bowel.

Symptoms include: fatigue; migraines; irritable bowel syndrome; inflammatory bowel disease; gallbladder disease; arthritis; asthma; rhinitis; recurrent infections; enuresis (bed wetting); attention deficit and hyperactivity disorder; epilepsy; eczema; psoriasis; aphthous ulcers (in mouth); and also reactive hypoglycemia.

You see these symptoms are common in the population and they are chronic, so to look for a cause of these symptoms is not what most of doctors do.

To see a psoriasis patient completely free of lesions after one month of stopping all cereals, flour, and pasta because of a suspected hidden allergy to wheat is fantastic. It encourages me as a doctor to look for the cause of the symptoms listed above.

There are at least two types of allergies and probably more. The first is the Type 1 hypersensitivity reaction mediated by immunoglobulin E (igE). It is quite a fast reaction and people realize right away that they are allergic to something.

The second type is the hidden or masked food allergy. Reaction is delayed and therefore difficult to associate with the food that is to blame for the symptoms. And most of the time, the allergic patient is addicted to the food that caused the problems. Why addicted? Because any allergy exposure provokes a release of cortisone by the adrenal gland and that cortisone, when it reaches the brain, is a feel-good hormone that gives a spike of energy.

So if you have any of the symptoms listed at the beginning of this chapter, try to find the food that you eat every day and the ones that you like the most.

Most of the time it did start in childhood and the symptoms are: colic; recurrent ear nose and throat infections; running nose; growing bone pains; asthma; eczema; and feeling sick all the time.

On examination, you will have pallor of the nasal mucosa and swelling dark circles under the eyes. You can become allergic or intolerant to a food just by eating too much of it. So having a diversified diet is a good thing.

The food that is the cause of the allergy or intolerance can be anything. The most frequent are: wheat; dairy products; all food that contains refined sugar; corn; egg; citrus fruit; coffee; tea; alcohol; food additives; and others.

How to make a diagnosis?

This is not easy because of the diagnostic tests: the scratch test (scratch on skin); the rast (R.A.S.T.) test (blood test); and the ALCAT test (blood test). They all have their advantages, but this means that sometimes they can find the food allergy, but sometimes they cannot.

So the best way is to find the allergy yourself by trying to stop eating different foods for at least a week, up to a month. The most frequent are flour (wheat) and dairy products. In the wheat, the allergen part is the protein gluten. In the dairy, the allergen is the protein casein.

Why are we more allergic now than before to those two proteins—gluten and casein? The answer may be because of heavy metal intoxication (mainly lead, mercury, cadmium, and others). The enzymes that we need to digest these proteins are affected by the heavy metals that bind to them and make the enzymes less efficient to digest the gluten and casein. When not completely digested, gluten and casein have the potential to become allergens.

When you have a food allergy (immediate or hidden), the lining of your intestine is swollen and that means that the natural barrier of your intestine lining is not doing its job. Digestion is a process where we cut food in very little pieces before they can be absorbed through the lining of intestines. The intestine lining is not supposed to absorb big undigested pieces. That means that only the very small pieces (the ones that are not allergenic) can get through.

But when the intestines are swollen (leaky gut) because of an allergy, the intestine may absorb pieces that are big (too big). Those big pieces of not completely digested food, when they get inside the blood, have the potential to create another allergy. So the problem of one allergy can create other allergies. I hope you see the picture.

Food allergy is an important part of looking for and understanding how to achieve optimal function of the human physiology. If you are allergic to a food, stop eating that food for the rest of your life. Suspected food can be stopped one type at a time.

The diet for the very, very allergic (and very motivated), who want to stop every food and then try to reintroduced the food items one by one, is called a highly restrictive diet. On this diet, you eat only lamb, pears, and spring water for five days and then reintroduce the other foods slowly, according to the symptoms. After a while, you may notice that you may eat the allergic food items once in a while without symptoms. This phenomenon has been reported. You will also notice that by stopping an allergy food, you may become less allergic to others.

Patients with hypothyroidism and hypoadrenalism have more allergy symptoms. So be sure that your thyroid and cortisone hormones are in the optimal range.

Food allergies are common. Look for the food you eat every day that you think you cannot live without. Then stop them one at the time for, let's say, one week and watch what happens. This will tag a food allergy that you may have without knowing it before. It also has the advantage of making you try other foods in order to have a more diversified diet.

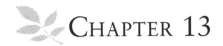

CHAPTER 13

Gout

Hyperuricemia

Gout affects many people who suffer acute attacks of arthritis, mostly in the big toe and also in the foot, ankle, and knee. The acute attacks are usually so severe the patient will look for medical advice.

When the diagnosis of gouty arthritis is made, the standard treatment is nonsteroidal, anti-inflammatory drugs for the acute phase and then a drug called Allopurinol as a preventive measure to reduce production of uric acid in your body. The high uric acid feels like grains of sand in your joints. This is the cause of gout. If you take Allopurinol for the rest of your life, the chances of relapse of acute gouty arthritis are reduced.

Are you interested in knowing why the uric acid is high in your body before you take a medication for the rest of your life? The cause of high uric acid is the food you eat that causes high insulin secretion. This means your body is intolerant to those foods and reacts by producing too much uric acid.

The solution I think is to stop eating the food that is poisoning you instead of taking a medication. Because by treating the cause (stopping the poisoning), you will heal the gout and all the other diseases that are associated with gout, such as metabolic syndrome (a prediabetic state), diabetes, obesity, high blood pressure, bad lipids, higher risk of bone marrow cancer, and alcoholism.

The cure is to stop eating the quickly absorbed glucides (carbohydrates).

Fast absorbed glucides (carbohydrates) include the following:

Sweet liquids, juice, adding sugar to coffee or tea, and beer

Bread, cereal (whole grain or not), flour, pasta, pastries, etc.

Rice (brown, white or yellow)

Potatoes of any kind

Desserts (all sweet things)

Your life will change radically because when you have gout you are already intoxicated by those foods. It is not just the spikes of arthritis. It is your whole system that is sick.

Most people will choose to take the medication (Allopurinol) rather than change their lifestyle. I understand this. They think that the problem is only the acute arthritis. But now you have learned that arthritis is only the tip of the iceberg. The iceberg is the metabolic syndrome of prediabetes, diabetes, high blood pressure, bad lipids, the risk of bone marrow cancer, alcoholism and other complications from these diseases. It is a never-ending story of complications.

So stop eating sugar and the things that are quickly transformed into sugar in your stomach. Your insulin (inflammatory hormone secreted by the pancreas) will be lowered, gout will stop (uric acid lowered), diabetes will stop, blood pressure will be normalized, chances of cancer will be lowered, and yes, the chances of heart attack and stroke will be lowered.

Can it be that simple? Yes, because it is basic physiology.

Now that you know the cause of gout, will you try to reduce the bad food you eat and do what works all the time—stop eating all bad food permanently?

CHAPTER 14

Restless Leg Syndrome

Restless leg syndrome affects too many people. Known to be family related, many people complain about it, but the standard medical treatment does not seem to be good enough. This syndrome is a discomfort in the legs, accompanied by a strong urge to move. The movement relieves the symptoms, but they recur with subsequent inactivity. Symptoms occur mostly in the evening or at night.

Some people have a lighter form. They have mainly cramps in their legs in the evening or at night, but this is not family related. This condition is mostly caused by a magnesium deficiency. It is corrected by magnesium supplements (magnesium citrate 300 mg twice a day). For family-related, restless leg syndrome, magnesium supplements will help, but it is not enough.

First: iron deficiency increases the symptoms. Ask your doctor to check your ferritin. It should be higher than 50 and under 100. Normal ferritin is usually

81

higher than 15. But for a restless leg syndrome patient, studies show that higher than 50 helps with symptoms. If your ferritin is lower than 50, you should take iron supplements until your ferritin gets to over 50 and under 100 (ng/ml).

Second, take a magnesium supplement (if you don't have kidney insufficiency): magnesium oxide 500 mg twice a day; and magnesium citrate 300 mg twice a day.

Magnesium is not a medication. It is food for your body. But, it will improve the symptoms only if you are deficient in magnesium. Magnesium is 10 times more abundant inside the cells compared to the serum. If you test the serum, it will be normal most of the time even if you have an intracellular deficiency.

The test to have done is called *Inside Red Cells Magnesium*. In one study of cardiology patients by Dr. Steven Sinatra, MD, Cardiologist, 75% of people tested were deficient in magnesium inside the cells. Magnesium deficiency is frequent and the symptoms are leg cramps at night.

If you have a kidney insufficiency, you lose the capacity to excrete the magnesium. By taking a supplement, magnesium could accumulate in your body, so check with your doctor.

Third, take melatonin nighttime supplements. Restless leg patients are known to produce less melatonin—a hormone secreted in the brain at night. Melatonin dosage: 0.5-1.0 mg before sleep.

Fourth, take folate supplements (probably faulty folic acid metabolism conversion to folate): folate 0.8 mg per day.

Folate is a better form to take because it is a ready-to-use vitamin by the body compared to folic acid, which has to be transformed to folate by an enzyme in your body before becoming the active form, which is folate.

Fifth, take a supplement of vitamin E (complete alpha, beta, delta, gamma) of Tocopherol and Tocotrienol. Mix vitamin E (the 4 tocopherol + the 4 tocotrienol).

You can find vitamin E complete at Life Extension (www.lef.org) or any good supplement shop. All this will help you a lot, but if not enough, you can add the standard medications, such as Mirapex, Requip, Neurontin, Lyrica, Opioid or Benzodiazepine. These need a doctor's prescription.

Summary of Suppliments

1. Ferritine: 50-100 mg/ml
2. Magnesium Supp. mg oxide 500 mg twice daily or Magnesium Citrate/300 mg twice daily
3. Melatonin: 0.5-1.0 mg nighttime
4. Folate: 0.8 mg per day
5. Vitamin E Complete: 1 per day

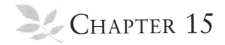

CHAPTER 15

Actual Medicine

(God help me for this one)

The role and responsibility of doctors is to help patients the best they can. To achieve that goal, doctors are trained in medical school by other doctors, PhDs and scientists. Lately, we have seen plenty of different fields in medicine developing—naturopathic, intregrative, acupuncture, etc.

I think that medical doctors are losing the global vision. That is the reason why all the other fields around medicine are developing to catch up on what doctors are missing. What is the global vision that doctors should have? When there is a mechanical breakdown, the good mechanic will find the cause of the problem in order to solve the problem for good.

But the cause of a disease is never a lack of medication.

Doctors in medical school are mostly trained at using medications when they diagnose a health problem. Doctors do their best, but it is difficult to learn all there

85

is to learn about medications and side effects, etc. By using medications (drugs) the patient does not really improve because the cause of the problem is still there.

So it is that simple. The global vision that all health care professional should have is to look at a problem with a vision of what is happening inside the patient, the science, and the physiology that lead to the problem. This means not just prescribing a medication that will only improve the symptoms, leaving the cause of the problem in place.

Doctors really do believe that they have been taught well at medical school. Since doctors are responsible people, they think that their fellow teachers will not fail in their responsibility of teaching what there is to know about human machinery breakdown. But they have failed them.

First, let's say that a lot of the causes of diseases are known—written in books, on the web and taught by organizations like the ACAM (American College for Advancement in Medicine), Functional Medicine.org, A4M (American Academy of Anti Aging Medicine), AGEMED.org and others.

So why is all that science not taught by the medical faculties? I've heard answers like, "We are so busy with the actual curriculum we cannot add more." I also think that it is a question of philosophy. The doctors who are in charge of medical faculties think it is the way to go because they have been trained like that and repeat the same mistakes.

And the doctors like me, who have been trained in both the medication system and the "find the cause" system, do not yet have the power to convince and to guide others in the right direction.

Today, patients still trust their doctors, but they ask more because they are educated and they read. Often they are more informed than their doctor about preventive medicine, bioidentical hormonal supplementation, nutritional medicine, supplements, diet, intoxication, and food allergies. By the way, these are subjects they do not teach in medical school.

Doctors like to get results. For me, it is more important than the pay.

Since I practice the "find the cause" approach and "prevent the problem," the results with my patients are better than expected—better than I or the patient expected. It is very rewarding and easy because it works.

I said that it is the responsibility of medical faculties to train doctors, but it is also the responsibility of every doctor to train himself and when trained—then train others.

I would like to talk about belief and science. Many doctors will say "I believe." Science is not about belief. Science is about knowledge. You know or you don't know.

Doctors are taught by scientists but often are not scientists themselves. It is the reason they like to "believe," because it is easier to believe than to do the whole process of learning the physiology in order to understand and then say, "I know!"

I did write this in the hope that everybody concerned with health care will be inclined to take on responsibility—including the medical schools, the doctors, all health care professionals, and not the least the politicians and voters.

Leaders have a big responsibility too. They listen too much to some lobbies and they hold with a leash the good doctors who want to innovate, to improve. We all have a responsibility.

Medicine is a science, so let's learn the facts and science about the causes and symptoms of diseases.

CHAPTER 16

Hormones (Endocrine)

Hormones are molecules made by glands within your body. They are sent into the blood circulation and then reach a specific receptor where they bind. This binding gives the message to the site of the receptor. So hormones are messengers in the machine. The human machine needs hormones to function properly at the right timing and in the right quantity. Hormones work together like a symphony. Their level should be optimal for the machine to work optimally.

That means that hormones cannot be said to be in the "normal range," like other blood tests. They have to be in the "optimal" range. For example, if your car tire pressure optimum is 35 psi in a blood test equivalent, the normal range would be from around 25 psi to 40 psi, but the optimum is 35 psi. You should inflate your tires to 35 psi to be at the optimum. Usually for hormones to be in the upper third of the normal range is optimal.

The causes of hormonal dysfunction include aging, autoimmune disease, toxic influences such as heavy metals and pesticides, and others. The solution to hormonal dysfunction is hormonal replacement, for now. In the future, maybe we will be able to repair the damaged gland with stem cells or other techniques.

This means if a hormone in your system is low and you have the symptoms of that low hormone, you should have that same identical hormone supplemented in the right quantity. This is called bioidentical hormone replacement.

One way to check is to look at Internet web sites that have questionnaires for hormone deficiency diagnosis. They are quite good because hormone deficiency symptoms are so obvious. Then, find a doctor who is trained in diagnosing and treating hormonal deficiencies. You can find them listed under associations such as the American Academy of Anti-Aging Medicine or the American College for Advancement of Medicine. Life Extension (www.lef.org) can help too.

The symptoms of hormonal deficiency are felt all over the body. When a hormone has receptors in brain cells, heart cells, skin cells, or muscle cells, the symptoms of that low hormone will be felt in all the cells that are lacking that hormone.

Why use only bioidentical hormones for replacement? The hormonal system is very intricate. Hormones are produced in glands, then they are sent to receptors where they execute their function. After that, they are removed and have to be taken out of the body.

All this has to work like a symphony. The same molecule used to replace the molecules you are lacking have a better chance to do the same job.

The principal hormones can be evaluated (blood tested and/or questionnaire), and supplemented when needed. These include: thyroid; melatonin; growth hormone; cortisol; DHEA; pregnenolone; aldosterone; estrogen (estradiol, estriol); testosterone (men and women); progesterone (women and men); and insulin. This last one must be kept low (middle third of normal).

When all your hormones are at an optimum level, all the cells of your body have a better chance to work at their optimum level. This includes your stem cells. More on this in the stem cell chapter.

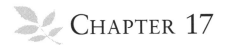

CHAPTER 17

Thyroid Hormone

The thyroid gland is located in the front of the neck. It secretes the thyroid hormone through the blood circulation. Then the thyroid hormone reaches its receptors in every cell, every nucleus, every mitochondria of the body. The quantity of the production of the thyroid is controlled by the pituitary gland (in the head). When there is deregulation of the thyroid production, the effect will be felt in every cell, meaning you are going to feel something.

Too much thyroid hormone production (hyperthyroidism) brings symptoms of fatigue, increased appetite, weight loss, anxiety, agitation, insomnia, and others. This is a serious condition. It should be taken care by a doctor who is experienced in treating hyperthyroidism. It is not common but the diagnosis and treatment of that disease is not the focus of this book.

Now let's talk about a too low production of thyroid hormone (hypothyroidism). This is very common. Some say that up to 40% of the world population has symptoms of hypothyroidism.

There are many ways to diagnose low thyroid functioning. A blood test will tell you the level of hormones but will not tell you if those hormones are doing their job, that is if they connect to the receptors or if receptors are healthy, etc. Basal temperature and Achilles tendon reflex are good ways to evaluate thyroid function. Basal temperature (taken in the morning when you wake up) should be higher than 96.8 F and lower than 97.7 F; or higher than 36.0 C and lower than 36.5 C.

The symptoms of low thyroid are: cold intolerance (cold hands and feet); fatigue (mostly morning activities); dry skin; constipation; obesity (difficulty losing weight when dieting); swelling all over (swollen eyelids, swollen calves); hoarse morning voice; morning depression; orange coloration of the sole of the foot; follicular keratosis (like goose bumps on the triceps' skin, back of arm); slow pulse rate; high diastolic blood pressure; small difference between systolic and diastolic blood pressure (usual difference is 40 mm hg; lower than 35 is a sign of low thyroid); slow Achilles tendon reflexes; slow thinking; poor concentration; faint heart sounds; muscle and articular pains; and depression.

You see, with all those symptoms you will notice that something is wrong if you have them. What is interesting is the diversity of the symptoms that are all over the body—brain, muscles (including heart), joints, blood vessels, skin, and soft tissue under the skin.

The thyroid hormone is needed throughout the body. What is interesting too is that if you get the appropriate treatment, all, and I mean all the symptoms, will disappear.

Let's look at why hypothyroidism happens. One reason is pituitary malfunction caused by radiation therapy for cancer or other pituitary dysfunction. Another is thyroid gland malfunction, caused by autoimmunity, pesticide intoxication, or fluoride intoxication.

Other causes include bad hormone metabolism (T4 should be changed to T3 in the right amount in the tissues) and bad receptors intoxicated by pesticides or fluoride. There are probably other causes that we do not know about. The best treatment would be to treat the cause. But to remove pesticides or fluoride from your body is another subject.

Be sure you have enough selenium (to change T4 to T3 (the effective hormone T3 is made by a seleno protein), enough zinc, enough iodine (to displace the fluoride), and enough vitamin D (for receptor binding).

Suggested supplements include:

Selenium: 100 microgram/day
Zinc: 25 milligram/day
Iodine: 1-2 milligram/day
Vitamin D3: 2000 international units/day

The usual treatment is to take thyroid hormone supplements.

Some say that taking T4 (Synthroid) alone is acceptable because your body should make the T3 it needs. In studies, around 33% of patients find relief from their symptoms by taking Synthroid (thyroxine T4), so 66% do not really get well. (*Hormone Handbook*, Thierry Hertoghe, MD),

For example, when you take Synthroid (T4 only), your blood test will become normal. But the symptoms of hypothyroidism may not completely go away if your body does not transform enough of the T4 hormone to the T3 hormone. T3 is the hormone that binds the receptor and does the job. T4 is the reservoir hormone and does need to be transformed into T3.

Because it is from the pig but it is close to human, the bioidentical thyroid replacement is a desiccated pig extract thyroid supplement (armour thyroid). It contains the right amount of T4 (80%) and T3 (20%) and most patients get relief from their hypothyroidism symptoms.

With desiccated thyroid pig extract, most patients receive a good blood test and relief of their hypothyroid symptoms. Because it contains the right amount of T4 and T3, it will be effective whether your ability to transform T4 to T3 is good or not.

If you have hypothyroidism, the other gland that may have problems is the adrenal gland (the gland that produces the cortisone). There is a high correlation between the two glands' dysfunction. And if you take thyroid supplements, it will make more work for the adrenal gland to produce more cortisone. If the adrenal is weak or sick, it will not be able to increase the production of cortisol. You will feel more tired. Cortisone is like the oil in the machine. If you add more thyroid, you will need more cortisone.

This means if you are going to take thyroid hormonal supplements, find a doctor who understands how your hormones are related and how they work together. That's the solution for optimum thyroid hormonal supplementation.

In all the hormone deficiencies, the thyroid is the most important to correct in order to relieve suffering. Do not forget to supplement cortisone as well, if you are deficient.

Some people will have the symptoms of a low thyroid, but blood tests can be normal. This may be what it is called hypothyroidism type 2. This is a resistance to thyroid hormone because the receptors for thyroid hormones are not working. This is explained in the book by *Hypothyroidism, Type 2*, by Dr. Mark Star, MD.

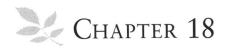

CHAPTER 18

Melatonin Hormone

Melatonin is a hormone that is secreted by the pineal gland (in the brain) during the sleeping hours. It is also secreted by the intestinal tract during the daytime. Melatonin is a guide for day and night hormone cycles (circadian). For example, this cycle consists of lower cortisol at night, higher growth hormone at night, higher thyroid T3 in the morning and so on.

Melatonin is secreted in the brain only when it is dark. So to have optimum natural secretion of melatonin, it should be very dark where you sleep or you should wear a sleep mask.

People who secrete enough melatonin look younger than their age, have less cancer and less neurodegenerative problems with aging, such as Parkinson's, Alzheimer's and dementia. For example, nurses who work the night shift are known to have more breast cancer. We believe this is because of lower production of melatonin when they sleep during the day.

So night-shift workers should sleep in a dark room or wear a sleep mask when they sleep and take melatonin supplements if they have any of the symptoms listed below. A blood test does not help to find out if you need melatonin supplementation, so we have to question the patient.

People who do not produce enough melatonin at night have a tendency for:

Agitation at night (easily woken up); restless legs syndrome at night; premature aging as adults; tired look (in the morning); poor dreaming; high blood pressure; seasonal affective disorder (winter or spring); anxiety; lack of serenity; and more intestinal cramps.

If you have any of the symptoms on that list, I recommend you try melatonin supplements, which can be bought without a prescription at your pharmacy or health store. The recommended dosage is from 0.5 mg to 3.0 mg taken at night. If you take too much, you will dream too much and you can wake up too early or too late. The ideal dosage is 0.5 mg to 1.0 mg.

The 3.0 mg dosage is for jet lag. You take 3 mg of melatonin at night for the number of days equivalent to the jet lag hours. For example, if you travel to Europe, you have a seven-hour time difference. In this case, you take the melatonin (3 mg) for seven days. After which, you come back to your former dosage which was from 0.5 mg to 1.0 mg.

Melatonin is a bioidentical hormone and can be bought without a prescription. Like any other bioidentical hormone, it is not dangerous and not toxic. Your body knows what to do with it in terms of metabolism and excretion.

But prescription or non-prescription hormones (all hormones) should be adjusted to their optimum amount. Hormones work together like a symphony and some hormones influence the behavior of other hormones. In the hormone world, do not take too much of a good thing because you will lose the benefits.

CHAPTER 19

Growth Hormone

It is called growth hormone because children who do not produce enough of this hormone do not grow. The growth hormone is secreted in the blood from the pituitary gland in the brain, mostly at night in men. Women secrete it mostly at night, but some during the day as well.

Children produce seven times the amount of growth hormone than an adult. In the adult, the growth hormone is needed at one-seventh the level of the children. At that level, the growth hormone is not needed for growth but for repair.

Growth hormone's utility in the adult is for repair and maintenance. So low growth hormone will lead to lack of maintenance in your body. Lack of maintenance in your body leads to premature aging. If you look at the symptoms of normal aging, they look similar to growth hormone deficiency.

Growth hormone can be measured in the blood by checking the "igf 1" or the insulin growth factor 1. The normal range is 114 to 492 ug/l, which is much too wide a range. The optimal level is in the upper third of that range. For men, 300 to 350 is optimal. For woman, 220 to 300 is optimal. For men, 0 to 250 levels are probably deficient. For women, 0 to 180 levels are probably deficient.

Some people will connect "growth" in the name of the growth hormone with cancer growth, but this is an association of the mind. There is no scientific proof of cancer increase associated with the replacement of growth hormone (up to optimal level) for somebody who was deficient.

In studies*, the replacement of growth hormones to optimal levels for people who were deficient reduced overall cancer by 40%. This was by taking growth hormone alone. If you take the right amount of vitamin D (2000-5000 iu/day), iodine (1 mg/day), selenium (100 mcg/day), and zinc (20 mg/day), your chances of developing cancer are reduced.

And cancer does not need growth hormone to grow. Cancer cells already grow quickly with or without growth hormone. But your immune system needs growth hormones to function properly and protect your body against cancer cells that may have started to develop. Most cancers happen at an age when people are deficient in growth hormone.

The symptoms of low growth hormone are: drooping

eyelids; prolonged skin fold after pinching the skin at the back of the hand for more than four seconds; prematurely aged body; hunchback; fat deposit above the knees; muscular atrophy of the foot soles which leads to pain when walking some distance; lack of inner peace; chronic anxiety without a reason; tendency to be depressed; lack of self control; tendency to social isolation; impaired social status; exhaustion with poor recovery; difficulty in recovering after not getting enough sleep; and, an excessive need for sleep.

Those symptoms are quite common in the population. They look like normal aging and they are. This is because they are caused by a reduced level of repair or maintenance, which is what we call normal aging. Most people older than 35 years do not have the optimal level of growth hormone and they age normally.

Simply put, if you are growth-hormone deficient as an adult and you take supplementation to bring your growth hormone to optimal levels, you will not age normally. This means you will still age, but you will feel and behave a lot younger. And the symptoms listed above will be significantly reduced.

Growth hormone is a bioidentical hormone, meaning it is exactly the same as what your body produces. It is a big molecule of 191 amino acids meant to be injected through the skin into the belly fat, exactly like people who inject insulin. The cost is around $200 to $500 a month.

One theory why growth hormone works so well is

that growth hormones help maintain and guide the stem cells we have naturally in every tissue, mixed with normal cells. These stem cells were thought to be "sleeping," but now we think that they are very active at maintaining and repairing the body as normal maintenance.

When we optimize all the hormones to their optimal levels, all the cells function better, but also the stem cells and that is a big step forward in understanding how reestablishing the body to optimal physiology will help the body heal itself.

Since it is a repair hormone, growth hormone supplementation will show its effects in two to three months and improvements will continue for around two years and after you are stable.

You can increase your own growth hormone production by: sleeping enough (8 hours); exercising; taking L-glutamine supplements (3 grams at night); eating the Paleolithic diet; eating organic food; and, staying lean because obesity is a state of growth-hormone resistance.

One glass of red wine with a meal is fine, but you should avoid alcohol, sugar, and anything that creates high insulin secretion, such as bread, yogurt, or milk.

Some say that growth hormone secretagogue can improve the level of GH (growth hormone). A secretagogue is less expensive than GH, which can be taken by mouth or as a nasal spray. You don't need an injection.

The pituitary gland, which makes the GH, has a

reserve of around three months of growth hormone. Secretagogues that increase the release of that hormone will work at increasing the GH for around three months. After that, I am not sure that they continue to offer any benefit. The natural way to increase GH production is to optimize the other hormones, such as testosterone, thyroid, melatonin, and estrogen (for women).

*Furstenberger G, Senn HJ. Insulin growth factors and cancer. Lancet Oncol. 2002 May;3(5):298-302.

Stoll BA. Breast cancer: further metabolic-endocrine risk markers? Br J Cancer. 1997;769(12) 1652-4.

Susan E Hankinson, et al. Circulating levels of insulin-like growth factor 1 and risk of breast cancer. Lancet. 1998 May 9;351(9113):1393-6.

Pratt SE, Pollak MN. Insulin like binding protein 3 (IGFBP-3) inhibits estrogen-stimulated breast cancer cell proliferation. Biochem Biophys Res Commun. 1994 Jan 14;198(1)292-7.

Marid O, et al. Growth hormone protects against radiotherapy-induced cell death. Eur J Endocrinol. 2002 Oct;147(4):535-41.

Crist DM, Kraner JC. Supplemental growth hormone increases the tumor cytotoxicity activity of natural killer cells in healthy adults with normal growth hormone secretion. Metabolism. 1990 Dec;49(12):1320-4.

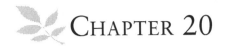

CHAPTER 20

Cortisone

Cortisone or cortisol is produced by the external part (cortex) of the adrenal gland just over the kidney. That adrenal gland cortex also produces aldosterone, DHEA, progesterone, and pregnenolone.

Cortisol is the only hormone that, if you do not have any, you die at the first stress on the body such as an infection. You need it for mood enhancement, dynamism, work capacity, stress resistance, stimulation of the immune defense, anti-rheumatic action, and anti-pain action.

Cortisone slows down the activity of the sympathetic autonomic nervous system, which brings calmness. So, if cortisol production is too low, you will have symptoms such as too much sympathetic action (too much adrenalin), armpit sweating, anxiety, sharp verbal retorts, nervousness, and irritability.

Cortisone is produced by the adrenal gland on demand by the pituitary. The pituitary sends ACTH (Adreno Cortico Thrope Hormone) into the blood. ACTH reaches the adrenal cortex and the adrenals hormones (cortisone, DHEA, aldosterone, pregnenolone) will be produced and released into the blood to create the actions at every cell that has a receptor for it.

Where does it lead?

Cortisone is the hormone needed for handling STRESS, so if there is a lot of stress there is a PRIORITY hormone production to produce more cortisol and less of the others (aldosterone, DHEA, pregnolone). This is called pregnenolone steal. This will work for a certain time because cortisol is a catabolic hormone (meaning it deconstructs or breaks down the body, lowers muscle mass, lowers bone mass), and it needs its compensating hormones like DHEA, which is anabolic (construct the body, increases muscles, increases bone mass, increases brain cell resistance to cortisol action).

So in a long, stressful situation, your body adapts in a way that helps you survive the acute phase by producing more cortisol but less DHEA. Most people are not made to resist stress for long. One test is to check DHEA with a blood test. If DHEA is low, pregnenolone steal is happening and you are already on the downward slope (high cortisol, low DHEA).

Stress can be good and fun if you have a proper level of cortisol and DHEA. But, as soon the level of stress you are comfortable with is surpassed, the DHEA production will be lowered in order to maintain cortisone production (pregnenolone steal).

This will work for a while but your body will be in a catabolic state (not good). Catabolic state (destruction state) can be seen as a cortisol dominance. The cortisol level is normally high but the compensating DHEA hormone is low.

This leads to post-traumatic stress syndrome, depression, and high cholesterol.

Why high cholesterol?

Because when the body sees a low production of DHEA, pregnenolone and aldosterone (these are steroid hormones, meaning made from cholesterol), the body tries to repair itself by telling the liver to make more cholesterol. That is the building block of the steroid hormone, which is lacking because the adrenal is so busy making only cortisone to survive the stressful situation. High cholesterol is associated with disease. But I think it is the low DHEA and pregnenolone that causes the problem, not the cholesterol.

Cholesterol is produced by the liver as the building blocks for steroid hormones (cortisol, testosterone, estrogen, DHEA, aldosterone and pregnenolone). Cholesterol is important for the proper function of the body. One of the best predictive tests of mortality at 70 years of age is low cholesterol. This means that over 70, if you have low cholesterol, your chances of dying early are increased.

While the body was succeeding at maintaining the

level of cortisone, the next step is adrenal burnout. The adrenal can no longer secrete the level of cortisol appropriate to the level of stress. That means your blood level of cortisol is in the low normal range in the morning, but you cannot increase it to a level sufficient to face the usual stress in your life.

Your symptoms will be:

A tired look; inflamed conjunctiva; sun tanning easily; running nose; allergies; salty food cravings; wet palms; irritable behavior; no patience; inflamed joints; abdominal pains; intolerance to medication; and insomnia.

Why insomnia? Because when the body is trying to make enough cortisone, the cycle of cortisol (low at night, high in the morning, medium in afternoon) may be lost and cortisol may be too high at night and prevent sleeping.

This is called borderline adrenal insufficiency. Your doctor will do tests and tell you your blood level of cortisol is normal and that it is all in your head.

The normal range for total cortisol at 8 h am (276-690 nmol/L). The optimal number is 550 nmol/L. If you are lower than 360 nmol/L, you are probably deficient in cortisol production if you have the symptoms of low cortisol.

Yes, the problem is in your head—and in every cell

of your body that does not have enough cortisone to function at optimum levels. The solution is to first try to reduce the stressful situation you are in (psychological and physical activities like exercising too much in evening). Eat a Paleolithic diet that keeps insulin low and eat enough fat for steroid hormone production.

Expose your eyes to bright sunlight in the morning, which increases cortisol release instantly. Sleep in a dark room, which keeps cortisol levels low at night. Save cortisol for the daytime.

Take supplements of B vitamins (complex—all B's), vitamin C 1000 mg twice a day, magnesium 500 mg/a day, omega-3 (EPA 1000 mg + DHA 500 mg/day). They help adrenal functions.

If all this is not enough, then find a doctor who knows about adrenal support and adrenal hormone replacement. The basics of all this are well explained in these books:

- William Jefferies MD, Endocrinologist, *The Safe Use of Cortisol.*
- *The Hormone Hand Book* by Thierry Hertoghe MD, probably the best hormone doctor, explains all there is to know.
- *Hormone Optimization in Preventive/Regenerative Medicine,* by Ron Rothenberg MD and Kris Hart MN, FPN, RN-C explains the philosophy and methods of hormonal replacement.

If you already have a diagnosis of hypothyroidia (low thyroid), your chances of having low adrenal function are increased. In fact, there is a strong association, maybe because the causative factors are the same.

When I started my medical practice 31 years ago, we would see 15 times fewer patients with thyroid problems. Thyroid problems are easy to diagnose and treat. There are 15 times more cases now compared to 30 years ago.

I think that borderline adrenal insufficiency is becoming very common and this a big challenge for doctors because the diagnosis is difficult. It requires blood tests and optimal results should be looked for (not normals).

The cause of the problem is probably the pollution. The world is a soup that we all live in. All the pesticides, chemicals, and heavy metals that are in the environment are in our body. The toxicity of one does not add up to the other—it multiplies it!

The glands in our body are hard working cells. They are sensitive to the intoxication of pollution. A great mind once told me: "A healthy human does not exist any more on this planet." When you take cortisone as a supplement (in physiologic doses) or as a medication (in a dose higher than the natural production), you should take at least a physiologic dose of DHEA (15 mg/day for woman, 25 mg/day for men) at the same time. Then the side effects that come from cortisol dominance will be avoided. This is important.

People who have adrenal insufficiency do suffer a lot. They live like there is a constant threat. They are not calm.

They experience reality as being more NEGATIVE than it really is for others. They feel good when on a relaxed vacation. Sometimes they will make dramatic changes in their life to reduce stress and enjoy life as much as they can.

There is a lot more to say about cortisol and how to cope with the world as it is. This is enough for now.

You can learn a lot more on this subject now that you have been introduced to it. My wish after this chapter is that people and doctors will understand that their symptoms of difficulty coping in the world we are in may be caused by hormonal dysfunction and can be treated successfully by hormonal replacement.

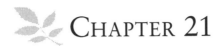

CHAPTER 21

DHEA
(DeHydroEpiAndrosterone)

DHEA is the most plentiful steroid hormone in the human body. It is made in the adrenal gland, in the same tissues that make cortisone, and it is made in the brain too. Cortisone and DHEA need to be secreted together for optimum physiology.

Some say that there is no specific DHEA receptor. DHEA probably has its effect by being a reservoir hormone and, when it gets inside a cell, the enzymes inside the cell changes the DHEA into the other hormones: androstenedione; testosterone; and estradiol.

Women get their testosterone mostly from the DHEA they produce in their adrenals. Most people over 40 years of age do not have optimum DHEA and by 70, the level of production of DHEA is very low.

Many bad things happen when DHEA is low: cognitive dysfunction; immune dysfunction (auto-immune); cancer; inflammatory diseases; cardio and vascular diseases; fatigue; depression; anxiety; low resistance to stress; low sexual desire; decreased erection (men); low sexual satisfaction (women); dry eyes; dry skin; reduced muscles; reduced axillary and pubic hair; reduced pubic fat; high cholesterol; and osteoporosis (weak bones).

You see all these symptoms are not specific. They look like normal aging and normal aging is what happens when our hormones get low over time.

People who have hirsutism (too much hair on face or skin) or acne probably have high DHEA.

Before buying DHEA that you can get over the counter, it is always better to have your blood level checked first. The optimal level is at the upper third of the normal level.

> ### Check the DHEA Sulfate:
> Women normal (1.3-9.8 ng/ml) Optimal = 7, probably low (0-4)
> Men normal (1.8 -12.5 ng/ml) Optimal = 9, probably low (0-6)

The recommended dosage for women is 5-25 mg (15 mg), one pill per day in the morning. The recommended dosage for men is 25-50mg (25 mg), one pill per day in the morning.

If you take too much DHEA, your nose will become oily and you may have acne. This is the same as when your DHEA was naturally high in the teenage years.

Any stressful event may reduce the production of

DHEA: pregnancies; loss of a loved one; etc. In order to maintain the supply of cortisone (the stress hormone), the adrenal gland will reduce the production of DHEA. This is a normal phenomenon, called pregnenolone steal, which happens in most stressful situations that last long enough to overwhelm the adaptation capability.

The stress situation provokes a catabolic (unbuild) state—too much cortisone (unbuild) and not enough DHEA (building hormone). The body can handle stress for a short time, but as soon as the DHEA is low, you are failing to handle stress.

So, if you feel stressed and have some symptoms on the list, have your DHEA checked. If it is low, take a supplement of DHEA: 15 mg (women) or 25 mg (men).

This may sound simple and it is. Since DHEA is a very important steroid hormone, its deficiency will create many symptoms that can be corrected by a simple supplement of the real thing—the real thing that is missing.

The philosophy with this is, if you have symptoms of low DHEA (most people over 40), your DHEA check is low. If you take DHEA supplements, most of the symptoms are corrected. If some symptoms are not corrected, then they were not caused by DHEA deficiency. Then you can look for other causes such as other deficiencies, heavy metal intoxication, bad food, etc.

An important thing to remember is if you take any cortisone prescribed by your doctor for an inflammatory condition, (asthma, rheumatoid arthritis, lupus, wegener, etc.), then you should take a supplement of DHEA. This is because when you take a cortisone supplement, it shuts down the production of DHEA by the adrenal and then you become automatically deficient in DHEA because you take cortisone. So cortisone and DHEA should be balanced so they work together.

But not the other way around. If you take DHEA supplements, it will not reduce your production of cortisone.

CHAPTER 22

Pregnenolone

Pregnenolone is the first steroid hormone made from cholesterol by an enzymatic reaction (P450 —Cytochrome) in the mitochondria of the cells of the adrenal cortex and in the brain. The two roles of pregnenolone are to be a precursor for the other steroid hormones (glucocorticoid, mineral steroids, androgens, estrogens), and second, pregnenolone is a neurotransmitter in the brain where it initiates the memory storage process by stimulating the enzyme adenylate cyclase.

Pregnenolone levels can be tested in the blood. The optimum level is like the other steroid hormones—the upper third of the normal range. When you test the pregnenolone sulfate, the normal range is 125-380 nmol/L, optimal = 285-315. People who are lower than 220 are probably deficient.

I think that patients with familial hypercholesterol should be tested for pregnenolone sulfate and, if low, be treated with pregnenolone supplements because low pregnenolone is a cause of high cholesterol.

The low production of all the steroid hormones happens when the enzyme P450 (making pregnenolone from cholesterol) is a slow worker in the mitochondria. This provokes a reaction by the liver to increase its production of cholesterol in order to have all the building blocks (cholesterol) needed to make the pregnenolone, which is the first in the production chain of steroid hormones.

The symptoms of low pregnenolone are: poor memory; reduced color vision; reduce artistic awareness; reduced sebum production (dry skin); and some joint and muscle pain. But it gets more complicated if pregnenolone is very low because the symptoms will be caused by the lack of all the steroid hormones.

The dosage of pregnenolone supplement is: physiologic (same as your body used to produce) 10-50 mg/ day. For memory enhancement, take up to 50 mg twice per day. The effect on memory does not last 24 hours if taken once per day. The symptom of too much pegnenolone is oily skin. Importantly, this looks like too much DHEA.

You are realizing that there are many things to worry about inside your body that need to be adjusted, leveled, and fine-tuned. Those hormones are molecules that belong to your body and your whole system will function better when these hormones are at their optimum levels.

Do we age because our hormones are lower or do our hormones get lower because we age? No matter what— get them adjusted and you will feel the difference.

CHAPTER 23

Aldosterone

Aldosterone is another steroid hormone secreted by the adrenal cortex. Its deficiency leads to symptoms of: low blood pressure; drowsiness when standing; eyes deep in orbit; and thirst that leads to frequent runs to the toilet during the day. But most important is the loss of hearing with age that can be caused by low aldosterone.

Aldosterone can be measured in the blood after standing and some activity. The optimum is in the upper half of the normal range. The normal range is 111-831 pmol/ml; the optimum is 415-831. Lower than 277 is probably deficient.

The standard treatment for aldosterone deficiency is fludrocortisone, a synthetic version that has the advantage of lasting 24 hours. The recommended dosage is 100 micrograms per day. But the real thing (bioidentical aldosterone) can be better at helping your hearing. The recommended dosage is 125 micrograms per day.

Too much aldosterone can make your feet swell and result in high blood pressure. Be sure to get enough potassium, from fruits for example, or lower the dose. Aldosterone (125 mcg/day) must to be taken for three months before hearing is improved.

I do think aldosterone should rarely be replaced only in exceptional cases. I am giving you the information because who else will?

CHAPTER 24

Estrogen

When you hear estrogen, you may be afraid of cancer? The only cancer that estrogen can provoke is cancer of the uterus if estrogen is given alone without progesterone. This also can happen naturally in the body of obese or premenopausal women.

When women stop ovulating, this means not enough production of progesterone in the second part of menstrual cycle, which leads to estrogen dominance. This leads to too much stimulation of the endometrium (cells lining the inside of uterus), which increases the chance of cancer developing.

Estrogens are three hormones that your body needs to function properly. What we should be afraid of is too much estrogen in obese or premenopausal women. The goal here is to have optimal estrogen and progesterone levels for optimal physiology (function of human body).

The estrogens are: estrone—called E1; estradiol—called E2; and estriol—called E3. The most powerful is E2 estradiol. It has receptors in the bladder, bones, arteries, vagina, heart, liver, and brain.

The symptoms of low estradiol are: persistent fatigue and depression; poor libido or sex drive; poor memory; hot flashes; night sweats; droopy breasts; vaginal dryness; weak bones (osteoporosis); and a pale face.

The least powerful estrogen is E3 estriol. Its effects are mostly that it thickens and humidifies the mucous membranes of the vagina, bladder, and eyes, maintaining their resistance to infection. Estriol has little effect on the endometrium and uterus. So the symptoms of low estriol E3 are dry eyes, itchy vagina, and frequent urine infections.

Estrone E1 is an estrogen hormone that does not need to be replaced because the body can make its own estrone from other estrogen.

If you are a menopausal woman with symptoms of low estrogens, the best way to have your estrogen hormones optimally replaced is with a trans dermal or trans mucosal (vulvar) cream called Biest. It contains E2 estradiol 20% and E3 estriol 80%. A dosage of 2.5 mg in 1 ml of cream per day applied to the skin of the inner arms or on the vulva (for better absorption) is a good start.

Note: With estrogen replacement, progesterone should always be prescribed as well. Progesterone can be put in cream in a dosage of 50-100 mg per day or progesterone can be taken by mouth. The pill is called Prometrium. They come in 100 mg and are bioidentical progesterone too. Bioidentical mean the exact same hormone that your body used to produce so it will have the same effect and the same elimination pathways.

By the way, the bioidentical hormones do not increase the risk of cancer.

Why not take estrogen by mouth like Premarin and other estrogen pills? Because, when taken orally, the estrogen will go to the liver first and the liver will react by increasing the coagulation factors. The risk of heart attack and stroke will be increased. This action of the liver (increasing coagulation factors) does not happen with progesterone or DHEA is taken by mouth.

So why are so many women afraid of estrogen replacement at menopause? Why are so many doctors afraid to prescribe hormones for menopausal symptoms? Why are so many women suffering from low estrogen at menopause?

In a Women's Health Initiative (WHI) study, the hormone Provera (medroxyprogesterone) was proven to increase the risk of breast cancer. So after that study, there was much confusion about all hormones. The purpose of the WHI was to study the non-bioidentical hormones Premarin (estrogen from horse urine) and Provera (a synthetic progestative), which is not bioidentical to progesterone.

The study on menopausal woman proved two bad things:

1. Provera increased the risk of breast cancer.

2. Premarin taken by the mouth increased the risk of heart attack and stroke.

But the study also proved that Premarin was good for bones, colon cancer, and cognitive function. So even if Premarin is made from horse urine, it could have advantages if taken in a transdermal cream to avoid passage through the liver and to avoid the increased risk of stroke and heart attacks.

All this should lead to the conclusion that the best way to optimize your body function is to have optimal hormone levels, good nutrition, exercise, ideal weight, and supplements like fish oil, vitamin D, vitamin C, a good multivitamin, magnesium, etc.

The hormones that were proven to be dangerous were not human-like hormones. Bioidentical human hormones are identical replacements for the missing hormones and there is no study (that I know of) that says that bioidentical hormones can be dangerous.

I remember a Honda car commercial that said, "Replace damaged parts with Honda original parts." So it is safer to copy nature, when it works so well. Doctors should learn to replace human hormones, when low, with identical human hormones.

Some say that if a woman has no uterus after a hysterectomy, when replacing hormones, she does not need progesterone to protect the uterus.

My answer is that all women have a brain and breasts and there are receptors for progesterone in the brain and breasts. So always take progesterone with estrogen when supplementing bioidentical hormones.

The effect of progesterone is not only to protect

from cancer. (There will be more in the progesterone chapter)

The ideal bioidentical hormone replacement for estrogen and progesterone is: Biest (estradiol 20% + estriol 80%) 2.5-5.0 mg per day in a transdermal cream; Progesterone (50-100 mg) /gram/day in a transdermal cream; or Prometrium 100 mg, 1 pill a day.

Men and Estrogen

The average man after 54 years of age has an estradiol level HIGHER than a woman of 54. That increase of estrogen in the aging man is caused by the enzyme called aromatase, which increases with the amount of fat.

Aromatase transforms the testosterone to estrogen, which is a lot more powerful hormone than testosterone, dose for dose. It tells the brain that there is enough hormone and the testicles will produce less testosterone. When this happens, men will have signs of low testosterone: weaker muscles; fat belly; fatigue; irritability; decreased libido; loss of drive and competitive edge.

Another sign of high estrogen is breast development. The diagnosis of this condition can be made by a blood test (estradiol, free testosterone, bioavailable testosterone). The treatment is first to have an ideal weight and exercise. An aromatase blocker (Arimidex 0.5 mg two times per week) can be prescribed to slow the transformation of testosterone to estrogen. This will increase the natural production of testosterone (more in the testosterone chapter).

CHAPTER 25

Progesterone For Women

Progesterone is the hormone that should always be prescribed when estrogen is taken. The reason is that any supplement of estrogen will lower the production of progesterone. Taking estrogen without progesterone creates estrogen dominance.

Estrogen dominance is a state of low progesterone with enough estrogen to bring symptoms of: anxiety; agitation; breast swelling and tenderness; bloating; fluid retention; headaches; mood swings; sleep disturbances; and heavy menstrual bleeding.

When a woman has these symptoms because of too much estrogen in her body and is not producing enough progesterone, mostly in the premenopausal years of 35 to 50, the simple replacement of progesterone will relieve all these symptoms.

Progesterone is produced in the adrenal gland (2 mg per day) of men and women. Before menopause in the second part of the cycle of women after ovulation, 20 to 40 mg of progesterone is produced by the ovary every day for 12 to14 days. So if a woman does not have an ovulation, the ovary will not produce the amount of progesterone (10 to 20 times more than the adrenal) that is needed to balance the estrogen already produced. This state of estrogen dominance will bring the symptoms listed above.

The simple treatment for that condition is to take a progesterone supplement half of the month during the second part of the cycle. If your period starts at the first of the month, you should take the progesterone from the 14th to the 28th day of the month. This means every month, all the time, until reaching menopause.

At menopause, what will happen is: you will have no more estrogen dominance because your ovaries will make less estrogen, your period will stop and then you will have symptoms of low estrogen or progesterone dominance (if you continue taking progesterone). Progesterone dominance brings mostly fatigue.

But low estrogen will bring symptoms such as: hot flashes; fatigue; decreased libido; urinary frequency; vaginal dryness; and weak bones. Then it will be time to start estrogen replacements to stop those symptoms, or it will be time to stop the progesterone supplements if you want no supplements at all.

This brings us to the subject of hormonal replacement after menopause.

The natural way for a woman to adapt after menopause is to gain some weight. Adding more fat to her body in the fat cells means the hormones DHEA and testosterone will be transformed to estrogen. This has the effect of raising the level of estrogen when a woman has more fat. Some woman will do well like that. Some will not.

The good effects of hormonal replacement are proven and have been experienced by women who have taken it. The bad effects are mostly fear of cancer. From what I know, and I did study a lot, there is NOT ONE STUDY that says bioidentical hormones increase the risk of cancer.

So we do not have enough studies to prove for sure that bioidentical hormones are 100% safe. My bias or educated guess is there are minuses and pluses in every decision for the average woman facing menopause without special cancer risk and the advantages win.

For a woman at menopause with an active cancer of the breast, ovary, or uterus, the fear that hormones will feed the cancer is on the mind of doctor and patient. But the scientific data on that subject are weak.

The hormones will help the immune system wage a better fight against the cancer and maybe the effect of the hormones on cancer cells will not make them grow faster. Also, we have to think of all the tissues that need estrogen to function at their optimum, like the brain. There are a lot of maybes. That is the reason why every patient's treatment should be individualized. The best decision should be taken according to the patient's needs, with all this guided by the best medical science.

I wish that doctors would learn the science of bioidentical hormone replacement. I wish that researchers looked at cancer and bioidentical hormone replacement.

Progesterone is safe to be taken at any age. During a pregnancy, the baby is flooded with 400 mg of progesterone produced by the placenta every day. That's 100 times the basic adrenal production.

Progesterone protects against cancer of the breast, uterine, and ovaries. It is the estrogen dominance that increases the risk of those cancers. Progesterone reduces the risk. So taking progesterone supplements when you have estrogen dominance is a very good thing to do.

Progesterone is a hormone naturally made by the human body. It is best to replace it with a bioidentical (exactly the same hormone molecule) sold in pharmacies.

I say that because there are patented hormones that are not bioidentical (not the same hormone molecule that the body makes) sold in pharmacies. Those that are not bioidentical are called progestins. They are not real progesterone. The best known is Provera (medroxyprogesterone) and it is known to increase the breast cancer risk in the WHI (Woman Health Initiative) study.

Progesterone can be taken by mouth. It is called Prometrium in pills of 100 mg with a dosage of 100-200 mg per day for the premenopausal woman taken during the last 14 days of the cycle.

For the menopausal woman, the dosage is 100 mg per day (27 days per month) for the woman who is also taking estrogen in a Biest (20% estradiol + 80% estriol) transdermal or transmucosal cream (2.5 mg per day).

Progesterone in cream (transdermal or transmucosal) with a dosage of 100 to 200 mg per day is for premenopausal woman when taken the last 14 days of her cycle.

Note: The progesterone cream can be mixed with the estrogen (Biest) cream.

Why take the hormones 27 days per month instead of all the time?

The answer is, in a petri dish, breast cancer cells die when you cut the supply of estrogen for five days. In real life, if we stop hormones for five days, many women have hot flashes, so we compromise at stopping for three days. You see this is not exact science. What we try to achieve is an improvement in the life of the patient taking into account all the factors that we can scientifically account for.

CHAPTER 26

Testosterone and Women

Women have testosterone too. In fact they have even more testosterone than they have estradiol, the main female hormone. Testosterone is very important for the behavior and the general look of a woman. The effect of testosterone is to maintain the mood, and reduce depression and anxiety.

It also maintains bone density, muscles size and strength, skin oil secretion, libido, sexual sensitivity, clitoris size and sensitivity, and orgasm.

It also protects against arteriosclerosis (cardiac and vascular diseases). In two studies (see References section), women with higher testosterone, DHEA, and androstenedione had less inflammation in the inside lining of carotid (neck) arteries.

A woman with low testosterone will be more passive and less inclined to do physical activity. Symptoms include low libido, less sexual satisfaction, fatigue, decreased muscle mass and power, depression, anxiety, memory loss, abdominal fat, weight gain, lack of self confidence, cellulite, varicose veins and fat accumulation in the breasts, abdomen, and hips.

Now I've got your attention and I think that no one wants to be low in testosterone.

Testosterone can be measured in the blood of woman as well:

Total testosterone: Normal (10-50 ng/ml)
Optimal 35 (0-25 probably deficient)
Free testosterone: Normal (2-15 pg/ml)
Optimal 8 (0-5 probably deficient)

The optimum is around the middle third of the normal range. The normal range is really too wide, so almost everybody would be considered normal even when they have symptoms of testosterone deficiency.

Your DHEA should be tested too because around one third of the testosterone of a woman comes from the conversion of DHEA into testosterone:

DHEA Normal (1.3-9.8 ng/ml) optimal 7 (0-4 probably deficient)

Taking birth control pills will lower the testosterone of any woman. This will not bother some because they had plenty of testosterone. But, for the women who were borderline low, taking a birth control pill could be dramatic. It will provoke the symptoms described before with the physical look of low testosterone: round back; small forward shoulders.

Eating cereals rich in fiber (whole grain bread, bran flakes) reduces testosterone by increasing the loss of testosterone in the stools. Much of the testosterone is secreted in the bile and thereafter reabsorbed in the gut and reused cereal fiber sticks to the testosterone and inhibits its reabsorption through the gut in the blood for a second use.

If fiber from cereals lowers the testosterone, the answer is to get fiber from vegetables. By not consuming cereals, flour, and pasta, you will lower your insulin level and increase your testosterone—two good things that have the effect of lowering inflammation, which is good.

Testosterone in a woman is produced in the ovaries and from the transformation of DHEA, made in the adrenal gland, into testosterone. Some testosterone is also made in the adrenal gland.

So when you make the ovaries rest by taking a birth control pill, the testosterone becomes lower. Then the woman depends more on the adrenal production and DHEA for her testosterone and sometimes this will not be enough testosterone production.

Women who have low testosterone should first treat the cause.

If it is because of birth control pills, then use another means of contraception that is not hormonal, such as a condom or intrauterine device with copper.

Consider not eating cereals, flour, and pasta.

DHEA levels start to go down after 25 years of age,

and after the stress of pregnancies. It is made in the adrenal gland, so any stress can reduce the production of DHEA. So if DHEA is low, an easy way to increase the testosterone is to take a DHEA supplement in a pill. The dosage is usually 15 to 25 mg per day.

If that is not good enough, a testosterone cream can be prescribed in a dosage of 1 to 10 mg per day. You see the range is wide from 1 mg up to 10 mg per day. This is because the sensitivity and metabolism of testosterone varies a lot. Every woman is different.

Is there a fear of body hair growth with testosterone supplements?

Body hair will grow too much when we supplement testosterone if we create a testosterone dominance over estrogen. If there is enough estrogen with testosterone, then body hair will not grow more. So in supplementing testosterone, we have to be sure that there is enough estrogen to begin with. If not, we have to supplement estrogen with the testosterone.

You start to understand that hormones work as a team. In every chapter, I try to describe each hormone individually. But in the real life, one patient will probably be deficient in many at different levels and when we supplement, we have to consider the sensitivity of the patient to each of the hormones. The personality and physical shape of a woman is very much influenced by testosterone—I think as much as men are!

CHAPTER 27

Testosterone In Men

The hormone testosterone has receptors in most tissues in the human body. That means that all the cells of human body need a sufficient level of testosterone to function properly.

Some of the important roles of testosterone are:

Safeguarding the cardiovascular system. Testosterone is needed for strong heart muscle cells. It widens the lumen of coronary arteries, minimizes arteriosclerosis, maintains normal blood pressure, and increases fibrinolytic activity (reducing blood clot formation).

Testosterone also protects against obesity and diabetes by reducing fat mass and increasing lean muscle mass and by increasing insulin efficacy to make glucose penetrate the target tissue of muscle, brain, heart, etc.

It supports the brain by increasing the blood supply and by increasing the connections between neurons. It increases the mood, memory, reduces anxiety, and maintains bone density.

The effect of testosterone is on all the tissue of the body. So everybody has a different setup of testosterone hormone level and receptor sensitivity to start with. That means that some men have a normal testosterone level during the teenage years. For some men, it will take a long time before they become deficient, by age 40, 50, 60, 70, and even 80. I have seen an 84 year old who was not deficient in testosterone.

But it also means that some men will always be deficient in testosterone in their teenage years. They will develop few sign of virilization such as sparse beard, poorly developed muscles, high tone of voice, few body hairs, etc.

But no matter how high your testosterone is when you are young, it will go down with the years. This is because of many reasons that we could understand better.

Pollution has an important role and is verified in young males in many mammalian species. Estrogen mimickers are many different molecules, such as pesticides and others that bind to our hormone receptors and poison our body. Heavy metals such as lead, mercury, cadmium, arsenic, etc., bind to enzymes that make our hormones. So those enzymes work less and our hormone levels get lower.

The cause of the problem should always be searched for. To avoid estrogen mimickers and heavy metals is difficult because they are in the environment. Drinking filtered water and eating organic food is a good start.

You have to be aware of the symptoms of low testosterone and then you will get immediate medical attention because I think that low testosterone is a medical emergency considering the bad things that happen to the body when in a low state of testosterone.

In the Archives of Internal Medicine 2006, men with low testosterone died 88% sooner than men with high testosterone. In Circulation (Khaw et al) showed that high endogenous testosterone was associated with lower mortality for cardiovascular disease and cancer. In fact, there is a 41% decrease in the chance of dying in men with testosterone levels of 564 ng/dl compared to a level of 350ng/dl and 350 ng/dl is not very low. I have seen many patients in the 180-200 level.

The consequences of low testosterone are:

- Cardiovascular system dysfunction that leads to heart attacks and strokes.
- Cognitive dysfunction, decreased memory, Alzheimer's and non-Alzheimer's dementia.
- More diabetes 2, dyslipidemia (bad lipids), osteoporosis, arthritis, and depression.

The symptoms of low testosterone are:

- Fatigue, depression, irritability (grumpy-old-man syndrome)
- Reduced sexual potency, desire, and fantasies
- Decreased morning erections
- Longer recovery time between orgasms
- Loss of drive and competitive edge

- Stiffness and pain in muscles and joints
- Decreased effectiveness of exercise workouts
- Pale face, lack of mental firmness, indecisiveness, hesitation.
- Abdominal obesity

If you have some of these symptoms, consult a doctor to check the blood level of testosterone.

Test:

- Free testosterone: N (5-25 ng/dl) optimum = (20-25 ng/dl)
  (0-18 ng/dl) probably deficient
- Total testosterone: N (300-1000 ng/dl) optimum = (700 ng/dl)
  (0-550 ng/dl) probably deficient.

When I said "probably deficient," it means that when the blood test is low, the symptoms of the patient have to fit with the blood result. Usually the symptoms of the patient will tell same thing as the blood tests. But if they are different, the patient's symptoms win.

Optimal range is a very important concept to understand. First, the normal range is established with statistics of two standard deviations over the average of 10,000 blood tests (not necessarily healthy) patients. This means that the top 2.5% have too high testosterone and the low 2.5% have too low testosterone. It also means that 95% of the people tested will have normal testosterone levels.

Now you understand why the "normal" levels should not be used. Instead, we should use the concept of "optimal," which corresponds to the level of testosterone—not too low, not too high—where the patient is free of symptoms.

The best reference book for optimum hormone levels that I know of is *The Hormone Handbook* written by Thierry Hertoghe, MD.

The facts about the fear of prostate cancer:

Prostate cancer is more frequent in patients with low testosterone. Some testosterone is needed to grow prostate cancer. But to add more testosterone will not make it grow faster. This is important.

Prostate cancer needs very little testosterone to grow. On a scale from 0 to 15, any level of testosterone higher than 2 will make the cancer grow, but 4 or 6 or 8 will not make it grow faster. This very important to understand because most of the men who have cancer of the prostate have a level of testosterone higher than 2. And if they received a supplement of testosterone, this will not make the cancer grow any faster than it is already is.

This is important to understand. If you do not have prostate cancer, the fear of developing it by taking a testosterone supplement is not justified. It is the opposite. Your risk of getting prostate cancer is higher when testosterone is low. If you already have prostate cancer, then you have to weigh the pluses and minuses. For example, if your cancer was operated on and is completely without metastasis and PSA (prostate specific antigen) is very low after two years, I think that your urologist will be happy to prescribe a testosterone supplement, if your testosterone is low of course.

If your cancer has a high Gleason score of 7 or 8 (aggressive cancer), you have bone metastasis and the best treatment is to keep the testosterone as low as possible, with a medication that stops production of testosterone. So, testosterone supplements are not for you except maybe at the end of life. A testosterone supplement is known to improve the quality of life because the low testosterone treatment that you were following is going to kill you too.

This is because the treatment of keeping testosterone very low for very aggressive prostate cancer slows down the cancer. But at the same time, it is causing very serious deprivation of testosterone in all the tissues of the body: brain tissues; muscles; joints, etc., and this has the potential to kill you before the cancer does. Testosterone supplementation (when deficient) should not be avoided on the unjustified fear of prostate cancer in the future.

Now you understand that it is important to take testosterone supplements as early possible after the diagnosis of testosterone deficiency is established. This will prevent inflammation in the vessels, brain, joints, and muscles and will prevent cancer of the prostate.

The means of testosterone supplements are:

Testosterone cream applied to the skin 50-100 mg/

day or testosterone subcutaneous self-injection 30-50 mg twice a week.

This usually corrects the problem. A blood test has to be done after a month to check the new level of testosterone and estradiol (estrogen). Estradiol should be checked because in some (mostly fat men), the testosterone will be transformed into estradiol. If this happens, a medication called Arimidex can be prescribed to block the enzyme aromatase, which transforms the testosterone to estrogen, and maintains estradiol at optimum levels (10-45 pg/ml, optimum 25, probaby too high >32).

The OPTIMUM concept applies to all the hormones in our body. All hormones have a function to do. Their optimum level is the level where the function is accomplished. Too low or too high will not do it.

We can picture it like the oil in your car. There is an optimum level and it is not a statistical measurement of the average 10,000 cars that enter the garage for an oil change. The optimum level of oil in your car is written on your oil gauge.

For humans, the optimum level of hormones is the level where there are no symptoms of deficiency and no symptoms of too much.

I wish you all a perfect level of testosterone!

CHAPTER 28

Contraception For Women

Contraception comes in many forms. If you use condoms or a barrier or copper intrauterine device, it will not change your physiology or behavior. This means you will remain yourself and your hormonal self will continue to work at what it was made for. This is because the condom, barrier, or intrauterine device with copper does not interact with your own hormones.

If you use a hormonal contraceptive, such as birth control pills, patch, or a hormonal intrauterine device (Mirena), it will change your body's hormone set up. This can change the way your brain works, your personality, and how you choose your mate.

First, let's understand how women are attracted to a man naturally.

Much of the attraction between sexes is chemically driven by pheromones (scent). This scent will help the woman decide which man she prefers. She will usually like the scent of an immune system of a man that is quite different from hers. So using the scent she prefers, she will choose the immune system of the mate. It is scientifically proven that couples with different immune systems will have children with stronger immunity (more resistant to infections).

Also, when a woman is ovulating, she has a spike of testosterone that influences the brain. She will be attracted by a more masculine, muscular man. She will dress to show more of her body. The spike of testosterone will make her body emit chemicals signals (pheromones) that show she is fertile.

When a woman takes a hormonal contraception that stops her ovulation (pill, patch, hormonal intrauterine device), the normal physiology is disturbed and it seems that a woman can choose a partner that is the opposite of what she would have chosen naturally.

Women who take hormonal contraception have a tendency to look for less masculine partners and to like the scent (pheromones) that is more in a category with an immune system closer to her own. So children born to a woman who was on the pill when she chooses her partner will have a weaker immune system.

What happens when a woman stops hormonal contraception? She may become more attracted to the more masculine male, mainly when she is fertile (ovulating). She may not be attracted anymore by the scent (pheromones) of the partner she has chosen while on the contraceptive.

On the man's side, the attraction of a man to a woman is chemical too.

The information a man gets when a women is fertile is through the scent and the look, mostly the waist-hip angles and straight shoulders (not hunched back).

Women on hormonal contraceptives have a reduced scent. They have lower testosterone that leads to less muscle power, which leads to a hunched back because the shoulders need muscles to fight gravity. The brain of a woman needs testosterone too to fight adversity; but this is another story. But generally, a woman on hormonal contraceptives will be less appealing to the males.

Hormonal contraceptives that interact with your own hormones are: pills; patches; and intrauterine devices with hormones in it (Mirena). Contraceptives that do not interact with your hormones are: condoms; barriers (diaphragms); and intrauterine devices with copper.

I think that relationships between men and women are complex and when you add a hormonal contraceptive into the equation you add to the complexity.

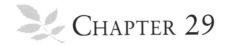

CHAPTER 29

Hormones

and Fear of Cancer

Hormones (the bioidentical ones—the exact same as your body produces) are part of the normal physiology. Having an optimal level of hormones is what is needed to have what is called HOMEOSTASIA. Homeostasis is a state of optimal function of the body and when there is optimal function—there is no cancer.

So does having balanced hormones lead to less cancer. Yes! So what are the unbalanced hormones that could increase cancer? The answer is high insulin, high estrogen unopposed by progesterone, low thyroid and low melatonin.

First, high **insulin** will increase the cancer risk because insulin is a growth factor for tumor cells. High insulin happens when you eat quickly absorbed glucides (carbohydrates), such as sugar, bread, pasta, potatoes, and sweet liquids. Insulin is secreted by the pancreas in order to lower the blood sugar because you have been eating bad sugar. Diabetes 2 is a state of constant high insulin and diabetes 2 increases the risk of ALL cancers. So, if you do not want to develop cancer, the first and best prevention is to eat a diet that keeps insulin low.

Second, high **estrogen** unopposed by progesterone happens to women who do not ovulate, mainly in their 40s. They have a tendency to be overweight with large and irregular periods. What happens is their endometrium (lining inside uterus) and their breasts are stimulated by their high estrogen production without the protection of the progesterone, which is naturally produced after ovulation.

This estrogen dominance state is also caused by a bad diet. Too much sugar maintains the high insulin and creates a state of high inflammation. This is interpreted as a disease state, which stops ovulation because it is not the time to make a baby. High insulin increases all cancers. High estrogen (unopposed by progesterone) or estrogen dominance will increase the risk of uterine, breast, lung and colon cancer—yes, lung and colon cancer are sensitive to estrogen dominance.

So for these women with high estrogen, high insulin, and low progesterone, to reduce their cancer risk means to eat a diet that keeps insulin low and take a supplement of progesterone (prometrium in pill form or a trans dermal cream of progesterone) during the second part of their cycle (from the 14th to 28th day of the menstrual cycle).

The other hormone that doctors and people like to

worry about is the **growth hormone.** And it is normal to worry about something that has a name like that because with cancer, what worries us is the GROWTH.

Growth hormone was named that because kids, who do not have enough growth hormone, do not grow. Let's look at dosage. Children's production and need of growth hormone is SEVEN times that of an adult. Yes, seven times. An adult produces seven times less growth hormone than a child. And in an adult, the normal or ideal production of growth hormone does not make anything grow. It does maintenance.

So in an adult, because of the quantity, the growth hormone should be renamed the "repair hormone" because that is what it does. Growth hormone at a level of 1/7th of the child's production does a maintenance job. It maintains our own stem cells' activity so they can nurture the cells around them and also divide when needed for repair and maintaining young-looking skin, young strong immune system, bones, heart muscle, etc.

To have a high igf-1 (insulin growth factor 1) is something that has been proven to increase the risk of cancer. High igf-1 happens when you eat improperly and have high insulin and also when you take growth hormone supplements.

When you take growth hormone supplements, you increase the igf-1, which promotes tumor growth, but you also increase the igf-bp3 (insulin growth factor binding protein 3) and this is a factor in fighting tumors. They balance each other in a way that patients who take growth hormone supplements have 40% less cancer in a study (see references in Chapter 17).

When a doctor prescribes growth hormone supplements, it is always in a state of igf-1 deficiency and the growth hormone supplement increases the igf-1 to an optimum level (men 300-350 ug/l, women 220-300 ug/l) and also increases the igf-bp3 to an optimum level (men and women 3000 ug/l).

Growth hormones also have cancer-fighting abilities of their own. They repair DNA (a cancer always has DNA damage). It increases natural killers such as white blood cells—first line of defense against cancer. It reduces Nuclear Factor Kappa B. This means more tumor cell death. It increases the production of vitamin D (good anti-cancer action). Supplementation for the deficient reduces visceral fat and insulin resistance, two things that were promoting cancer. So the hormone set up that promotes cancer is high insulin, high igf-1 and low igf-bp3.

When you take growth hormone supplements, you should have a diet that maintains a low level of insulin. So low insulin (igf-1 optimal) (igf-bp3 optimal) is the perfect setup to avoid cancer in the first place and to fight any active cancer because of a better immune system.

Thyroid

The other important hormone is thyroid. Low thyroid levels are known to increase the risk of all cancers. Low thyroid function is also associated with:

fatigue; cold intolerance; weight gain; dry skin; coarse hair; high cholesterol; increased severity of coronary artery disease; low mental clarity; and higher mortality among hospitalized patients.

Thyroid hormone, mostly the T3 (in the studies*), fights and prevents cancer in many ways. T3 increases the natural killer cell activity, white blood cells' line of defense against cancer.

T3 also increases the interleukin-2 receptors on monocytes, which is good. T3 decreases aromatase activity. Aromatase transforms most of the steroid hormones into estrogen. To have low T3 is bad for breast cancer risks.

T3 increases the oxytocin, a hormone that reduces the risk of breast cancer.

T3 and T4 both repair DNA as it comes under attack by free radicals.

There is an epidemic of hypothyroidism (low thyroid function) on this planet. In children, we see 30 times more than 30 years ago and for adults around 10 times more.

So if you want to prevent or treat cancer and improve your chances of not dying early from all causes, have your thyroid hormones checked and replaced at optimum level. If found to be not Optimum (that is: a TSH (Thyroid Stimulating Hormone) of 1 mu/ml and Free T3 in the low upper third of the Normal (FT3 Optimal=2.5-3.4 ng/l) Normal 1.8-3.7 ng/l. or (FT3 optimal=3.9-5.2 pmol/l) normal 2.8-5.7 pmol/l).

Melatonin

Women who work the night shift have lower melatonin production and have more breast cancer. How do you know if your melatonin is low? A blood test does not help. Melatonin is probably low if your dreams are few and when you are more tired and in a bad mood in the morning.

If you are deficient, melatonin supplements are a good means of preventing cancer and treating an active cancer. The dosage is 0.5-1.0 mg at nighttime in pill form.

Cancers develop in three stages: initiation; promotion; and progression:

Initiation is the DNA damage that is caused by radiation, free radicals, pesticides, solvents, plastic (toxic), or abnormal genes (mutation).

When a cell's DNA is cancerous, does that mean you will have cancer if the next steps fail? There are ways for the body to fight cancer: repair the damaged DNA—if it cannot repair, the cell should go in apoptosis (that is programmed cell death if it cannot repair itself). Also, the immune system with natural killer cells with Interleukin 2 should get rid of the offender.

Promotion is a period when the cancer cell makes a colony since they survived the body's effort to get rid of them at the beginning when they were few. They grow in a tissue by reproducing (dividing). At this time, the body's immune system has some time to win the war.

This period of promotion can last months (melanoma), to years (5-7 years for breast cancer).

Progression is when the cancer cells invade the body. It is also called metastasis. That means that you lost the war on the cancer cells.

Let's look at our subject of hormones and cancer. First, no hormone can initiate a cancer because no hormone has the capacity of doing DNA damage. Where hormones are involved is in the promotion phase.

"High insulin" hormone is a "growth factor" for cancer cells and it slows the activity of the immune system. High estrogen when "dominating" (not enough progesterone) will make estrogen-sensitive tissues (breast and endometrium) grow more and have an increased risk of cancer promotion and progression.

The other hormones (growth hormone, thyroid, melatonin) are there to improve the ability of the body to fight the cancer, so it is when they are too low that the cancer risk is increased.

To make myself clear, it is when your hormones are at an optimum level that the body is functioning at its best—less cancer, less chronic disease, etc.

Most hormones have to be checked and adjusted by your doctor. But the one that is the most damaging for cancer is insulin when high and it is easy to control it yourself by eating a diet with no quickly absorbed sugar (glucide).

Cancer is now the number one cause of death in America. When you drink a sweet liquid, eat flour (whole grain or not), eat potatoes (in large quantities), or anything that will increase the sugar in your blood, it is like buying a lottery ticket for cancer.

*Kmiec Z, Mysliwska J, Rachon D, Kotiarz G, Sworczak K, Mysliwski A. Natural killer activity and thyroid hormone levels in young and elderly persons. Gerontology. 2001 Sep-Oct;47(5):282-8

Balazs C, Leoey A, Szabo M, Bako G. Stimulating effect of triiodothyronine on cell-mediated immunity. Eur J Clin Pharmacol. 1980 Jan;17(1);19-23

CHAPTER 30

A Star of Medical Research

Now meet Dr. Bruce Ames, Emeritus Professor of Biochemistry and Molecular Biology at the University of California, Berkeley. His research looks for the mechanism of degenerative diseases, mitochondria decay, nutrient deficiencies, and DNA damage leading to cancer. Dr. Ames authored more than 500 research papers.

What follows is an abstract of an interview with Dr. Bruce Ames from Life Extension magazine, August 2011.

He reports that when he gave acetyl-L-carnitine and lipoic acid (two natural molecules that are reduced in our mitochondria when we age) to older rats, it did improve their mitochondrial function to more resemble the mitochondria of younger rats. The cognition (all brain activity, intelligence, memory) in these older rats got better and also in dogs when they are fed these substances.

That means that acetyl-L-carnitine and lipoic acid are supplements that work on rats and dogs. Also, any supplement that helps mitochondria functions should help all the organs that spend a lot of energy like the brain (cognition, Parkinson, Huntington) and the heart (cardiac insufficiency).

Dr. Ames's work suggests that if you're modestly deficient in one of the essential micronutrients, then your body has to ration them in terms of priority. Under this scenario, the body will direct nutrients toward short-term health and reproductive capabilities—and away from regulation, repair of cellular DNA and away from repairing proteins that increase longevity.

This means that while your body may be providing nutritional support in an effort to sustain system-wide physiological function and reproduction at the cellular level, the process of decay and death is accelerating if you are deficient in micronutrients.

How does this play out in real-world dietary terms?

To run your metabolism, you need the basic macronutrients of fuel, fats, and carbohydrates. You also need 15 or so vitamins that are co-enzymes and 15 or so minerals that are required for enzyme structure. Then you need two essential fatty acids, omega-3 and omega-6. That's roughly 40 substances that your body needs for optimal function.

Virtually every metabolic pathway requires micronutrients. Deficiencies in these micronutrients may NOT be severe enough to create immediate clinical symptoms, but the long-range implications could lead to an increased risk of disease associated with aging.

The work of a scientist, Jim MacGregor, showed that folic acid deficiency in mice and humans leads to the breakdown of chromosomes, just like radiation. According to his research, this occurs in 10% of the American population. This means a significant number of people are experiencing critical DNA damage without realizing it because they have a lack of folic acid in their diets. It is like being irradiated.

Based on this idea, Dr. Ames observed that whenever he made human cell cultures in a petri dish a little deficient in a vitamin or a mineral, they started to suffer DNA damage—not just deficiency in folic acid. Any other deficiency provoked DNA damage. This is very important because DNA damage is a serious cause of diseases like cancer.

Dr. Ames also worked on vitamin K. Known as the vitamin for coagulation, vitamin K is also known for its role in blood vessels and bones. Dr. Ames says, "In the United States, the population tends to be fairly low with regard to vitamin K intake, largely due to the fact that we do NOT consume sufficient greens. In Japan, people obtain healthy amounts of vitamin K from a soy product called Natto. We believe that Natto consumption may be responsible for the decreased risk of fractures and bone loss among Japanese women. Additionally, Natto may be responsible for the lower prevalence of arteriosclerosis (vascular disease) in Japan."

Concerning obesity, Dr. Bruce Ames said: "Obese people are hungry all the time because the body is craving missing nutrients such as magnesium. Sixty percent of the American population is too low in magnesium. Even though people are obese and look like they are well fed, they are basically starving for vitamins and minerals. According to a colleague of mine (Dr. Ames's colleague), Americans aren't getting enough fiber. On top of which, people are consuming vast amounts of simple sugar, which can poke holes in your gut. Bacteria are leaking, triggering inflammation. The purpose of a balanced diet is to get all your vitamins and minerals and we are not doing that."

The last subject is what Dr. Ames recommended to prevent cancer. Dr. Ames said to eat a good diet and do not smoke because smoking takes about 8 to 10 years off your life. And I think a bad diet takes off another 8 to 10 years of your life. You have to convince people that they're going to lead miserable lives if they get fat and spend years suffering from diabetes and their brains will be fogged. The choice seems obvious.

What impresses me the most is the scientific fact that, when human cells are deprived of the essential nutrients, they start to develop DNA damage, which is how cancer starts.

Also, what impresses me is the fact that old mitochondria can function like young mitochondria when supplemented with acetyl-L-carnitine and lipoic acid. Those two supplements are cheap to buy and are naturally produced in the body in bigger quantities when we are young.

The other important subject is vitamin K for bone and vascular health.

These are important scientific facts that advocate the importance of supplementing with vitamins and minerals, in addition to a good diet. That means a good diet is not enough.

Will you take the chance of missing just one of the minerals or vitamins when you know now that it can provoke DNA damage? Mostly, we know that the supplements at the recommended dose are safe. This means if you take a supplement you were not deficient in, then you take the supplement for nothing. You will not have side effects.

But before making any changes in your medication prescribed by your doctor, ask your doctor if the supplement negatively affects the medication.

When you take all the supplements, you make sure that your essential vitamins, minerals, and essential oils are in your body for optimal function.

It is also a fact that there are 50 enzymes that need vitamin B to function at optimum levels. When one or more of these enzyme levels start to become low, a supplement of B vitamins can repair the enzyme function.

That means that if all those enzymes are working well, you do not need vitamin B supplementation. But if just one of those 50 enzymes is low, you would benefit from vitamin B supplementation.

Clinically, it is difficult to measure enzyme activity. My advice is to give vitamin B supplementation to all my patients. To take 10 times the RDA (Recommended Daily Allowance) for vitamin B has no side effects. I said, "without side effects." The only change is you will have very yellow urine, which is the color of vitamin B2.

And with that amount of B vitamins, you will have the comfort of knowing you are not deficient in the B vitamins, which are important for metabolism of mitochondria and enzymes.

Some people still doubt the need for vitamin and mineral supplementation when eating a good diet. I hope that this chapter did convince you that there are no chances to take, because any deficiency of minerals, vitamins, or essential oil can have serious consequences.

Everyone wants to have a better life and extend their good days, so you should take supplements as insurance to be sure of not missing something.

The supplements that I recommend are:

A good multivitamin with minerals but without iron. They contain around 50 mg of each B vitamin with zinc 10 mg, selenium 100 mg, etc.

Vitamin C: 1000 mg twice per day

Magnesium: 500 mg per day

Vitamin D: 2000 iu per day

Fish oil: EPA 1000 mg - DHA 500 mg per day.

This is a good start!
If you want mitochondrial support you can add:
Acetyl-L-carnitine: 250 mg twice per day
Lipoic acid: 150 mg per day
CoQ10: 50 mg per day

For vitamin K supplementation, which helps to keep calcium in the bones and out of the blood vessels walls, I recommend:
Vitamin K 2: 1 mg/day
Vitamin K 1: 1-5 mg/day

Note: If you take anticoagulation medication (Coumadin), supplements of vitamin K are not recommended except in very low dosages. For example, vitamin K1 (1 mg/d) + vitamin K2 (0.2 mg/d) will have the effect of stabilizing the coagulation and stabilizing the dosage of Coumadin at a little higher rate than before. This means that if you take Coumadin—do not take supplements of vitamin K unless your dosages of Coumadin need to be changed all the time. Then a little supplement of vitamin K will stabilize the coagulation and the dosage of Coumadin. Talk to your doctor before changing).

Conclusion

This is a good base of supplements for most people. You can buy those at most health food stores or pharmacies. I like to think of the supplements as an insurance policy that prevents accidents!

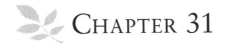

CHAPTER 31

Carnosine
(An Outstanding Supplement)

Carnosine is used for the prevention of Alzheimer's, arteriosclerosis, diabetic complications, near-sight vision, and cataracts. It is present in high concentration in the muscles and brains of many animals and humans.

A scientific paper written by Dr. Alan R. Hipkiss (London, England) from September, 1997, states that carnosine (B-Analyl-L-Histidine) has a protective function in addition to anti-oxidant and free-radical scavenging roles. Carnosine extends the life of human fibroblast cells in a petri dish culture (which is good). Carnosine kills transformed cells, which are cancerous and pre-cancerous cells (which is good).

Carnosine protects cells against aldehydes and amyloid peptide fragments (aldehydes and amyloids are very toxic to cells). Amyloids are the deposits in brain cells that we find in excess in Alzheimer's disease.

Carnosine inhibits in vitro (in the laboratory), the protein glycation formation of cross-linking carbonyl

AGE (Advance Glycation End Products) and DNA/protein cross-linking (protein that sticks to DNA by a sugar bond).

Glycation is one of the mechanisms of getting old. It happens when a molecule of sugar bonds with a protein. This makes the protein no longer usable for the body. That is why diabetics get old faster—high sugar makes more glycation.

Cross-linking is the same mechanism as glycation, but it involves two proteins that become bonded together by a molecule of sugar. This is very bad when glycation or cross-linking happen to our precious DNA.

Carnosine is a scavenger of lipofuscin, the colored stuff in skin age spots.

Because of all of these actions, carnosine is a possible modulator of Alzheimer's disease, arteriosclerosis, and diabetic complications.

If there was a medication (I mean a patented drug) that was that good, there would be a lot of sellers to explain the benefits and convince you to take that medication to prevent the most feared diseases of our times—Alzheimer's, arteriosclerosis, and complications of diabetes.

Carnosine is found naturally in high quantities in the muscles and brain cells of humans. With aging, that amount is reduced. By taking a supplement, you can increase the amount of carnosine in your body and potentially reduce the aging process, which is caused by glycation, cross-linking on our DNA and other proteins that our bodies need to function properly.

Another problem caused by glycation is presbitia, difficulty reading, which comes with aging. Most people after 45 years of age, will need glasses for near sight. Presbitia is caused by a glycation (sugar that sticks to protein) of the cristalin, the lens of the eye. Using drops of carnosine in the eye every day for life can reverse the problem.

Cataracts (opacification of the eye lens) are caused by glycation too.

So using carnosine eye drops every day may slow and even reverse the problem. Carnosine in pill form can be bought in any health food store. The dosage is 500-1000 mg twice per day.

The best way to get the most benefit from carnosine is to increase the dosage until side effects occur. One would be muscle twitching (one muscle that contracts every 5-10 seconds). When this happens, you reduce the dose to the maximum level when no muscle twitching occurs. Muscle twitching happens in the face, shoulders, or anywhere on the body.

Carnosine in eye drops is another story. There are many products but most give a sensation of eye irritation when used. One type that causes no eye burning sensation is Can-C eye drops made by www.profound-products. com. It is a 1% n-acetyl carnosine solution. The dosage is 1-2 drops two times per day.

There is no literature on the uses of carnosine as a supplement. My personal experience goes back to when

I was 42 years old, 13 years ago. I needed glasses for near vision and I decided to find out why my eye lens was no longer adjusting for near vision. I found that it was because of a glycation problem in the lens that had lost its elasticity. Then I read an article on carnosine (an anti-glycation molecule) that can fight glycation. Since that time, I have taken carnosine in pill form, 1000 mg, twice per day and one eye drop in each eye at nighttime. My near sight vision became normal after one month of using the carnosine. I did stop using carnosine for one month and the near sight vision problems started again. But after one week of carnosine supplementation, the problem was solved again.

The aging mechanism of glycation will always be there. When you age, your body produces less anti-glycation product or carnosine. When you decide to take supplements with carnosine, it has to be for a lifetime. This requires discipline. Some will prefer to age normally and this is their choice. But for the ones who are disciplined and willing to take charge of themselves, there are plenty of things to do in order not to age normally. After reading this book, I hope that you will have enough information to make choices.

CHAPTER 32

Vitamin A

Why include a chapter on vitamin A? Because you hear on the news that some vitamins can be toxic, like vitamin A at high dosage and vitamin E when supplemented with only alpha tocopherol and iron, when you have enough in your system.

Note: When supplementing with vitamin E, you should use a mixed tocopherol (4) and tocotrienol (4).

Vitamins belong in your body, which means you should have an optimum level so physiology function is at its optimum level. But do not use vitamin E (alpha-tocopherol) alone because it depletes the other vitamin E, mostly the gamma tocopherol.

The fat-soluble vitamins (A, D, E, K) can be toxic if you take too much because they have a tendency to accumulate in the fat. Usually toxicity comes after a long time of too much supplementation and mostly if you are old, have a liver disease, or are an alcoholic.

The other vitamins (B and C) are hydrosolubles (soluble in water). They cannot accumulate in the body so if you take too much, they are excreted by the kidneys in the urine. So theoretically, the water-soluble vitamins cannot bring toxicity in the event that you take too much.

Vitamin A should be at optimum levels. This is very important because optimum levels of vitamin A help to reduce the risk of: cardiovascular disease; cancer; age-related eye macular degeneration; and cataracts. Vitamin A, at optimum levels, also helps appropriate immune responses, which are very important in autoimmune and infectious diseases. Vitamin A is also needed for bone formation. Vitamin A deficiency in children is associated with iron deficiency, anemia, and poor growth.

The diagnosis of low vitamin A can be made by looking at the skin on the back of the arm (triceps) for goose bumps called hyperkeratosis. Also dry, cracked heels are a sign of vitamin A deficiency.

The New England Journal of Medicine, 1990 reports a study of children hospitalized with severe measles who were given 400,000 units of vitamin A. There was 75% reduction in mortality compared to those given a placebo (flour or sugar pills). That is an impressive result for just a vitamin. Others studies published in the American Medical Association Journal and British Medical Journal report similar results in children supplemented with vitamin A—a 39% reduction of death from diarrhea and 79% reduction death from measles.

Those studies did describe the use of vitamin A as if it were a medication. This means they did not test the level of vitamin A before they administered it.

The important fact is there was a very high increase in better health when vitamin A was given to a patient who was believed to be deficient. In that case, the children who had a tendency to become very sick from diarrhea or measles were probably deficient in vitamin A before they got the disease and it probably was because of this deficiency in vitamin A that they got very sick.

There are a lot of unknowns because these studies did not check the level of the vitamin A to see if the patients were deficient before being given the supplements of vitamin A.

That leads us to the point that when we give a patient a medication we do not check the level of that medication before because we know that it is none: there is no normal level of medication for optimal physiology. But for optimal physiology, everyone should have optimum levels of all the vitamins.

Some believe that when you eat right you should have enough of all the vitamins. But in science, I do not like beliefs—I like facts. In food, you get vitamin A from liver and eggs. Your body can also synthesize vitamin A from the carotenoids in oranges, fruits, and carrots. When you get older, the capacity to absorb vitamin A in the gut is reduced. When you are hypothyroid, your capacity to transform the carotenoid in foods to vitamin A is also reduced.

Some people have a genetic problem and cannot transform carotenoid into vitamin A. In one study in

England, 47% of women have this problem. People who cannot transform carotenoid from food into vitamin A because of low thyroid function or genetic problems will have an orange coloration of the soles of their feet.

What is the best thing to do? Should everybody be tested for levels of vitamin A? I do not know! But prevention is always better than treatment. This means don't wait to get a disease caused by a deficiency in vitamin A before taking supplements of vitamin A.

> Vitamin A deficiency can be very dangerous. Symptoms include chronic illnesses, autoimmune diseases, increased susceptibility to infections, hyperkeratosis, dry skin and increased cancer of the colon, lung, breast, and prostate.

In a Johns Hopkins School of Hygiene and Public Health report, it stated, "It is now estimated that improving the vitamin A status of all deficient children worldwide would prevent one to three million childhood deaths annually." My educated guess is everybody should take a supplement of vitamin A which is enough to compensate for any deficiency, but low enough to be sure that levels do not get near the toxic zone.

That dosage is 10,000 units of vitamin A per day. This amount is safe for all adults, including pregnant women, the old, those with liver disease, and alcoholics. For babies up to 2 years old, 1,500 units of vitamin A per day and for children 2 to 12 years old, 5,000 units of vitamin A per day is good.

When you take a supplement of vitamin A, I think it is also good to take a supplement of vitamin D because they compete for the same receptors in the gut. So a supplementation of one can deplete the other one if you take only one. I recommend for adults vitamin D supplements of 2000-5000 units per day; children 2-12 years of age 1000-2000 units per day; and for babies up to 2 years of age, 400-800 units per day.

* KP West Jr and Ian Darnton-Hill. Nutrition and Health In developing World, 2008.

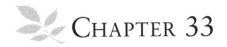

CHAPTER 33

Iron (too much)
Hemochromatosis

Too much iron in your body can be bad. People who take iron supplements when they do not need them, meaning they already have enough in their system, will have a shorter lifespan. Iron is essential for optimum physiology of the human body, so we should have enough, but not too much.

Some people have a tendency to be low in iron. They include children who grow quickly when they are young and woman who have excessive periods. They are easily identified by their doctors. They have iron deficiency anemia and can take iron supplements for treatment. The cause of the larger periods should be investigated and treated. The nutritional cause for the kids' iron deficiency should be investigated and corrected (mainly drinking too much milk).

People with a tendency to be high in iron have a disease called "hemochromatosis," a genetic, inherited disorder in which excessive amounts of iron accumulate in various tissues. Hemochromatosis is quite frequent in people of European descent. The symptoms of too much iron in tissues will be the failure of that organ when intoxicated with iron because iron is a powerful oxidant. This will happen with men in their 50's and women in their 60's. For women, this is because they are protected during their reproductive years when they lose blood every month with their periods. They lose the iron that is part of the hemoglobin in the blood.

The symptoms of too much iron or hemochromatosis are: liver disease; diabetes (pancreas and all mitochondria damage); joint pain (mostly knee cartilage); heart failure; fatigue (brain neurons and mitochondria); and erectile dysfunction (blood vessels and nerves). All those problems can lead to a shorter life.

Note: People with hemochromatosis are known to have low DHEA, probably from the toxic accumulation of iron in the adrenal gland where the DHEA is made. This may explain the low bone density and erectile dysfunction that is common in people with hemochromatosis. DHEA is an important steroid hormone for optimal physiology of human body. You will find more in the chapter on DHEA.

So, everybody should be tested for iron quantity in the body. The test is a blood test called "ferritin." The normal range is 24-336 microgram per liter(ug/L), but the optimum range is 50–100. That means people with a range under 50 may be ok, but if they have, for example, restless leg syndrome, the symptoms in their legs will improve if ferritin levels are kept between 50-100. For people who have a ferritin level higher than 100 ug/L, they have a tendency to accumulate too much iron. It may be they have the gene of hemochromatosis or maybe they absorb too much iron in their intestines for another reason.

Those with a ferritin level higher than 100 ug/L should never take iron as a supplement. They should donate blood regularly to keep their ferritin under 100 and over 50. When you donate blood, you lose iron. For every 500 cc (15 ounces) of blood given, the ferritin level goes down 75 ug/L, although it varies with patients.

You may read articles in newspapers that say supplements (multivitamins) can lead to a shorter lifespan. This is because "high iron" levels are common in the general population and if these people take a multivitamin that contains iron—that is a problem. It will reduce their lifespan, like people who have hemochromatosis. So my opinion is that a multivitamin with minerals should never contain iron. Iron should be taken as a supplement only when the patient's iron level has been proven to be low and the supplements should be stopped when the levels normalize (ferritin 50-100 ug/L).

Everybody should have ferritin tested in their blood as part of their annual checkup. Anyone with ferritin levels higher than 100 ug/L can donate blood regularly to keep their ferritin in the 50-100 ug/L range.

Homochromatosis is common (usually diagnosed

when ferritin is higher than 336 ug/l), but most people who have it do not know it, nor does their doctor. This is a condition that is very difficult to diagnose by the symptoms. So a simple ferritin test taken during your annual blood test can find out if you have accumulated too much iron.

You should ask your doctor for the results because, if your ferritin is in the normal range 24-336 ug/L, your doctor will see it as "normal" but "optimal" is different. Any patient with a ferritin level higher than 100 ug/L will benefit when the level is lowered to under 100 and over 50 ug/L.

Anyone who has a tendency to accumulate too much iron should limit their alcohol consumption because it increases the iron absorption and adds to the toxicity of iron in the tissues. To reduce the absorption of iron from the gut, black tea is known to be helpful in patients with hemochromatosis. It will reduce the amount of times you have to donate blood because the iron that you eat, mainly from red meat, will not be as easily absorbed from your intestine into your blood because it binds to the tannins in the black tea. The dosage is a cup of black tea at every meal.

You see there are a lot of things that people are willing to do to stay healthy. This chapter is about avoiding a toxin (iron). I think that by knowing your level of iron and maintaining the ferritin in the optimal range of 50-100 ug/L is a major step in the right direction to prevent problems.

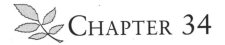

CHAPTER 34

Omega-3 (fatty acids) Some Facts

Omega-3 is a type of fat that is essential to the structure of all our cells' membranes, including those in the brain, muscles, blood vessels, kidney, liver, immune cells and so on.

If we get enough omega-3 in our food, then our cells' membranes get all the omega-3 fatty acids that are necessary for their construction and the functioning of those cells will be optimal. This seems simple. You should take omega-3 supplements to ensure the optimum physiology of all the cells in your body. So if you take a supplement of omega-3 and you notice an improvement, which means you were deficient in omega-3.

The point to understand here is you should not add more omega-3 to your diet than the body needs. You just take the amount of omega-3 that your body needs to stay at an optimal level.

Omega-3 helps conditions such as: depression; anxiety; cardio-vascular disease; cancer; premature death from all causes; attention deficit; and hyperactivity. These are conditions caused partly by a deficit in omega-3.

So by taking supplements of omega-3, you will help the condition by treating the cause.

If the lack of omega-3 was the only cause of those diseases, a supplement of omega-3 would cure 100% of them, but deficiency in omega-3 is only partly to blame for those conditions and other causes have to be looked into as well.

It is difficult to get enough omega-3 in the diet. The best way to be sure to get enough is to take it as a supplement. Fish oil is a good source of EPA (eicosapentaenoic acid) and DHA (docosahexaenoic acid). These are the long chain omega-3s that were used in most of the studies. The most impressive study was with the Inuit of Greenland in 1963. They got 80% of their calories from animal fat, fish, and seals (mostly raw). They were found to have no cardiovascular disease, no depression and no cognitive deficiency with aging.

Their diet was low in omega-6 (vegetable oils) and high in omega-3 (fish oils). They had a low inflammation diet, including low amounts of quickly absorbed glucides (low insulin); low omega-6 (low inflammation); high omega-3 (low inflammation); and, the animal fat they ate was uncooked—not transformed by high temperatures (low inflammation).

There are studies that say a lot of toxicity in the food, protein, fat and glucide comes from cooking at high temperatures—higher than boiling temperature of

220 F or 100C. You will find more information in the chapter on cooking.

Some facts:

People who have had a heart attack and had the highest level of omega-3 in their blood were found to have much lower cardiac arrhythmia (arterial fibrillation) and were prevented from dying of any cause by 85%.

A Norwegian study of men 64 to 76 years old who took supplements of 2.4 gr/day of omega-3 had a 47% reduction in the risk of dying from all causes.

An Australian dietary intake study on women found that those with the highest omega-3 consumption had a 44% reduction in risk of mortality from inflammatory diseases and the effects were dose related, meaning the more they took omega-3 the better.

A study of higher dietary intake of omega-3 is associated with a 34% reduction in the risk of symptomatic depression compared with people having the lowest rate of consumption of omega-3.

A study on a population of substance abusers demonstrated a reduction of anxious feelings when treated with 3 grams per day of omega-3.

People with the highest intake of omega-3 also have a 46% lower risk of metabolic syndrome (a pre-diabetic state).

Omega-3 reduces the risk of getting cancer and also reduces the risk of dying of a cancer. A study comparing the Mediterranean diet with an American

Heart Association diet found a 56% reduction in risk of developing a cancer and a 61% reduction in risk of dying from cancer in the Mediterranean diet group. Intake of omega-3 was higher in the Mediterranean diet group than the American Heart Association's recommended diet.

Men with the highest blood level of omega-3 have a 40% reduced risk of prostate cancer.

In a group of premenopausal women at high risk for breast cancer, those consuming the highest ratio of omega-3 (more fish oil) and less omega-6 (vegetable oil) had a 50% reduction of the risk of developing breast cancer.

People consuming the largest amount of omega-3 also had a 31% reduction in their risk of developing chronic kidney disease.

Kidney transplant recipients with a higher level of omega-3 in their blood had a lower risk of transplant rejection.

Risk of hospitalization for arterial fibrillation (a cardiac arrhythmia) is reduced by 81% in omega-3 supplemented patients.

Risk of depression and anxiety is reduced by 30% if you take omega-3 supplements.

Heart attack survivors will have an 85% reduction in the risk of dying from all causes if they take omega-3 supplements.

Breast cancer survivors will have 41% reduction in risk of dying of all causes if they take omega-3 supplements.

Hemodialysis patients will have a 57% reduction

in risk of dying of all causes when taking omega-3 supplements.

Men without cardiovascular disease will have a 47% reduction in risk of dying of all causes when supplemented with omega-3.

I hope you are happy with these numbers. They are impressive because rarely does a medical intervention have such efficiency. I think that omega-3 fats are needed in our body. If all the studies show such good results, it is because most people are deficient in omega-3. The easiest way to have enough omega-3 is to take a supplement of fish oil (long-chain omega-3).

Flax seed oil (short chain omega-3) can be used by people who are intolerant to fish oil, but most of the studies were made with long-chain omega-3 (fish oil).

> **Fish oil dosage recommendations (read the label) are:**
>
> EPA 1000 mg/per day (adults)
> DHA 500 mg/per day (adults)
> This means two to four capsules of fish oil per day.

I found studies in Dr. Alan Gaby's book on nutritional medicine that say omega-3 supplements help those with the following conditions:
- adult respiratory distress syndrome
- age-related macular degeneration
- angina

- ankylosing spondylitis
- anxiety
- aphthous ulcers
- arrhythmia
- asthma
- arteriosclerosis
- autism
- cancer
- Crohn's disease
- cystic fibrosis
- diabetes
- dysmenorrhea
- eczema
- dyspraxia
- hypertension
- IgA nephropathy
- kidney transplant
- liver transplant
- migraines
- night blindness
- pancreatitis
- photosensitivity
- psoriasis
- Raynaud's disease
- rheumatoid arthritis
- high triglycerides
- ulcerative colitis

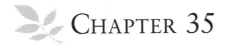

CHAPTER 35

Vitamin B-12 Deficiency
(More common than you think)

Vitamin B12 is needed for red blood cell production, nervous system function (mood and memory), and the immune system (allergies, autoimmunity).

The signs of a deficiency can differ among patients. These include: fatigue (chronic); weakness; concentration difficulties; pain; numbness and tingling of hands and feet; low back pain; arteriosclerosis (coronary heart disease); irritability; depression; confusion; memory loss; and dementia. That can be difficult to differentiate from Alzheimer's in the severe cases.

We get vitamin B12 from food, mainly meat, such as liver, kidney, chicken, fish, seafood, and eggs. Vitamin B12 needs to be separated from the protein that it is attached to in the meat to be absorbed into the bloodstream. This is done during normal digestion. When you age, low acid production in the stomach (achlorhydia) reduces the absorption of vitamin B12 from the food.

Other conditions that reduce vitamin B12 absorption from food (meat) are:

- All causes of low acid production in the stomach such as stomach surgery (for ulcer treatment), gastritis, medication that reduces acid production from the stomach (histamine 2 blockers—Zantac and others, The Proton Pump inhibitors—Prilosec and others.) Those conditions reduce the absorption of vitamin B12 from food only. They do not reduce absorption from vitamin B12 supplements because, in the supplement, the vitamin is free and not bonded to a protein.
- Aspirin—the mechanism is probably by damaging the gastric mucosa.
- Oral contraceptives (birth control pills).
- Metformin (a medication for diabetes).
- Helicobacter pylori (a bacteria that often lives in the stomach) causes low acid production.
- Vegetarianism (because of low access to vitamin B12) if patients do not take supplements of vitamin B12.
- Pernicious anemia.

There are many causes for vitamin B12 deficiency and it is becoming more common. The symptoms of vitamin B12 deficiency can be severe and very debilitating. The best way to diagnose vitamin B12 deficiency is to blood test everyone at their annual examination. This is easy to do. But the normal levels of the laboratory are not the optimum. Simply put, you should be in the upper half of the laboratory normal results.

Example 1 (for measurement in pmol/L): Vitamin B12 normal level is 185 to 630 pmol/L. The optimal is above 370 pmol/L. That means that if you are under 370 pmol/L, you are probably deficient in vitamin B12 and the optimum is around 520 pmol/L.

Example 2 (for measurement in ug/L): vitamin B12 normal is 250 to 850 ug/L. But the optimal is over 500 ug/L. That means if your level is under 500 ug/L, you are probably deficient in vitamin B12. The very optimum is around 700 ug/L.

Why does the lab not indicate the optimal level? In short, the goal of the lab is to find patients who are very low and have symptoms of the deficiency. All the others are considered normal. But life and science are not that simple and we have clinical evidence that some patients in the lower third of the normal range have symptoms of deficiency. Since vitamin B12 supplementation is very safe, it is better to have a level of vitamin B12 in the upper half of the normal range, where symptoms of deficiency are uncommon.

To supplement vitamin B12:

Pills: Methylcobalamin or Cyanocobalamin. The dosage is 1 mg per day. This equals 1000 micrograms per day.

Injections: B12 intramuscular. The dosage is 1 mg per

month. This equals a 1000 micrograms intramuscular injection every month.

No matter whether you use pills or injections, a blood test, after two or three months of treatment, will show if the blood level of vitamin B12 is up to the optimum and if the dosage needs to be adjusted. My experience shows that with pills of 1 mg per day (1000 mcg/day) of Cyanocobalmin or Methylcobalamin, the two kinds of vitamin B12, most patients are in the optimal range.

If you want to find the causes of diseases, you have to look for them. The cause of many symptoms that affect humans is often a deficiency in vitamin D, vitamin B12, and vitamin A.

CHAPTER 36

Iodine (Deficiency)

We know that iodine is added to salt, so is it something we should worry about? Iodine is not a medication. It is an atom in the family of halides (fluoride, chloride, bromide, iodine). Iodine is a very important factor in human physiology. In the 1920s, it was obvious that many people were suffering from low iodine in their food intake. The consequences were mental retardation, cretinism, low thyroid function, and goiter (big thyroid gland in the neck).

So a decision to add iodine to table salt was adopted and the rest is history. The people who were most affected by low iodine were the inland residents, because the ones living by the sea who ate fish and algae usually got enough iodine from seafood.

So why do we now have to worry about iodine again? Half of the salt consumed in USA does not have added iodine. Many people reduce their consumption of salt, for high blood pressure reasons and others and cooking with heat removes 65% of the iodine. The reason why Japanese women have less breast cancer than Americans is associated with the fact that Japanese women consume a lot more iodine in their diet, mainly from the algae that they eat as salads.

The fact that conditions like fibromyalgia and fibrocystic breast disease improve with iodine supplements is another clue that iodine deficiency is one of the causing factors in these diseases. Do we have a crisis of diseases caused partly by a deficiency in iodine? The answer is YES. Those diseases are: breast cancer; fibromyalgia; hypothyroidism; stomach cancer; obesity; cognitive impairment; psychiatric disorders; and chronic fatigue.

To make things more complicated, iodine is needed in the receptors of the steroid hormones in our body. If we lack iodine, even if we have normal levels of steroid hormones like estrogen, testosterone, progesterone, cortisone, DHEA, pregnenolone and aldosterone, the receptors lacking iodine will not work and your body will act like it has a deficiency of steroid hormones.

If the steroid hormone receptors that need iodine for their activities are intoxicated with other halides (mainly bromide or fluoride), those receptors will not work efficiently. The solution is to be sure to have enough iodine in your system to displace and excrete (in the urine) the fluoride and bromide. That means, since there is more fluoride and bromide in the environment, the solution is to get more iodine from food or supplements just to be sure that the iodine requirements of our body are met.

Recent studies say that 74% of the world population

may not consume enough iodine. So how much is enough? The RDA (recommended daily allowance) is 150-290 micrograms and the maximum is 1100 micrograms (1.1 milligram) per day. These guidelines were established as sufficient only to prevent goiter. In Japan, the average consumption of iodine is 5,000–12,000 micrograms per day (5-12 milligrams). In the treatment of fibrocystic breast disease, doses of iodine of 3,000-6,000 micrograms (3-6 milligram) per day have been used without side effects.

My recommendation is to take as a supplement of iodine 1,000 micrograms (1.0 milligram) per day and for the rest of your life.

For those interested in breast cancer prevention, there are four supplements that have been identified as reducing the incidence of breast cancer:

Vitamin D (2000–5000 international units per day).

Iodine (1.0 mg–12 mg per day) usually part iodine and part iodide.

Selenium (100–200 mcg per day) usually in a good multivitamin without iron.

Zinc (15–50 mg per day) usually in a good multivitamin without iron.

My recommendation is one milligram per day of iodine. But your doctor may recommend more, for a period of time, when treating a severe deficiency, until the deficiency is corrected. Then the one-milligram per day is a good maintenance dose.

The main cause of intelligence deficiency (low IQ)

in children on this planet is iodine deficiency. And the latest statistics say that 74% of the world's population does not consume enough iodine.

* Dunn, J.T., *Iodine, Modern Nutrition In Health and Disease*, Tenth Editon, Baltimore, MD; Lippincott Williams and Wilkins;2006:300-311.

* Nyenne, E.A., *Recognizing Iodine Deficiency In Iodine Replete Environments*. N Englang J Med; 2007;357:1263-1264.

CHAPTER 37

Dementia/Cognitive Decline/Alzheimer's

In a study of the Inuit of Greenland done in 1963, it was found that they did not suffer cognitive decline related to aging. The explanation comes from their diet: 80% of their calories come from animal fat, eaten mostly raw. An important part of this fat is from fish. They ate 20 times more fish oil than the American diet. So the question is, can Alzheimer's, Parkinson's disease, and vascular dementia be caused by a bad diet? The answer is YES!

The former diet of the Inuit has the physiologic advantage of keeping the hormone insulin low. I say former diet because the Inuit do not eat like their ancestors anymore. Now they eat pizza, drink sodas and cook their food at high temperatures like we do. Now they have the diseases of the industrialized world—diabetes, high blood pressure, etc. And the typical American diet, including flour (bread, pasta, cereals), sweet liquids, potatoes, rice and sugar, has the disadvantage of keeping insulin high.

Insulin is the AGING hormone. So, when you eat food that increases insulin production by your pancreas, you are going to age faster and develop the diseases of the old.

There are reversible causes of dementia, meaning they can be cured. They are:

Vitamin deficiencies—B12, B6, folic acid, thiamin B1, magnesium and iron. This occurs from poor diets, alcoholism, after stomach surgery, patients on diuretics and patients on long-term antacid medication.

Vitamins are absorbed through the gut. Foods need to be digested and this starts with acid in the stomach, which is needed to activate the enzymes made by the pancreas to digest the food. Not enough acid in the stomach will lead to food not being separated in small pieces and only small, digested pieces can be absorbed through the gut. Then the vitamins will go through the stools without being absorbed in the body. But if you take vitamins as a supplement, they are already in small pieces and they will be absorbed in your body.

Not enough iron can cause dementia, but too much iron can cause dementia as well. So iron must be optimized. You should have a blood test called ferritin and your level should be between 50-100 ug/L.

It is difficult to measure magnesium in the blood

because it is in the inside of the cells where magnesium is important. A good way to ascertain whether your magnesium is low is if you have muscle pain or cramps in the legs at bedtime. If you do, a magnesium supplement (magnesium citrate 300 mg at night) will get rid of the leg cramps and prevent dementia as well.

Vitamin B12, B6, B1, and folic acid can be measured in the blood. The optimal level is in the upper midrange of the normal range for those vitamins.

The second reversible cause is hypothyroidism. The thyroid gland function can be checked by a blood test easily done by your doctor.

The third reversible cause is prescription medications and over-the-counter medications. Many medications taken for chronic problems have a diminution of cognition as a side effect. Sometimes we think it is the disease or aging that makes the brain less efficient, but the medication can be a cause too. The best known are: statins (anti-cholesterol); beta blockers (heart and blood pressure); and, anti-cholinergic (allergies, over-active bladder). The best way to know if a medication is causing brain fog is to stop the medication for a short period. Be sure to ask your doctor first because, for example, it is dangerous to stop a beta blocker suddenly.

Most dementias are irreversible, such as Alzheimer's, Parkinson's, vascular (blood vessels blockage in the brain) and Huntington's (genetic).

Some dementias can be reversible, such as heavy metal intoxication (lead, mercury) and hormonal deficiencies (testosterone, estrogen, progesterone, thyroid, human growth hormone, DHEA, pregnenolone).

When the brain is foggy with low memory, reasoning, learning capacity and attention span, along with personality changes in mood and behavior, it happens for a reason. Your cells are alive, but not functioning well for a reason. If it is caused by low vitamins, low hormones or heavy metal intoxication, it can be repaired.

But there are situations where some of your brain cells have been amputated—they are basically dead. At the time of diagnosis of Alzheimer's, we think that half of the brain cells are already dead. So we look at irreversible dementia (cognitive decline) as an amputation of the brain cells. This happens over time. It starts in your 30s and is an inflammation process where all the bad things add up. These include a diet that creates high insulin, insufficient nutrients in your diet, smoking, alcohol abuse, heavy metal intoxication, and lack of exercise.

My recommendations to prevent damage to the brain and optimize the functioning of the cells that you have left include:

Exercise:

Studies say that exercise maintains brain circulation.

Healthy diet:

Keep insulin low by avoiding cereals, flour, bread, pasta, rice, potatoes, sweet liquids, vegetable oils (omega-6) and desserts. Recommended foods include vegetables, nuts, olive oil (omega-9), avocado (omega-9) along with meat, chicken, eggs, and fish, all organic if possible and cooked at low temperatures (under 250^0 F). High temperature cooking creates chemical reactions in the protein, sugar, and lipids, to a point where they become toxic. Remember, the early Inuit ate a lot of uncooked animal fat and they were very healthy.

Hormones:

Have your hormones replaced by bioidentical ones when they decline with advancing age. Some can be bought as supplements, others need a doctor's prescription and monitoring. These include: estradiol; estriol; testosterone; progesterone; DHEA; pregnenolone; thyroid; vitamin D3; melatonin; and human growth hormone.

Some people think there is a debate about the benefits of replacing hormones when they get low with aging, but it is clear in my mind that your body is made to function with an optimum level of hormones. When they are lower, a lot of symptoms of hormonal deficiencies start to appear and it is not nice. When you replace them with bioidenticals, you attain the same level of the same hormones that your body knows and used to be happy with.

Supplements:

Take supplements to ensure there is no deficiency of the nutrients that are known to be important for brain function.

Recommended supplements:

Multivitamins (with all the B vitamins, selenium, zinc, boron) but no iron, which should only be supplemented if you are deficient;
Omega-3 (fish oil EPA 1000 mg/day and DHA 500 mg/day);
Vitamin D3 (2000-5000 international units/day);
Coenzyme Q 10: (50-300 mg/day);
Vitamin C: (1000 mg twice per day).

To that list you can add some supplements that have great anti-inflammatory power. They are resveratrol (250-500 mg/day), pomegranate extract, acetyl-L-carnitine (500 mg twice per day) and alpha lipoic acid (150 mg twice per day).

Can we regrow the brain cells that we've lost? The answer is YES! But, we have to start early because they do not grow as fast as we would like. First stop the insults that kill your brain cells (eating bad food, etc.).

Progesterone is a hormone that is known to improve neurogenesis (growth of new cells) of brain cells.

Human growth hormone is a hormone that is known to maintain the stems cells that are needed to grow new cells (see chapter on growth hormone).

Some antidepression medications have the ability to increase the amount of brain cells.

Dementia is a bigger problem than we think. Some people do not develop their full brain potential because of chronic inflammation, even at a young age. This can be corrected by a simple diet adjustment. So many will suffer from dementia, it is easy to predict—just look around you at what people are eating and drinking.

If you don't want your brain to lose cells, then protect them and feed them real human food. Do not eat an inflammatory diet that will make your body fight the inflammation that destroys the most sensitive and precious cells of your body. Inflammation is sometimes needed for repair or fighting infections, but it is the chronic inflammation that we need to avoid.

There is a blood test that measures inflammation, CRP (C Reactive Protein) that is very precise. The optimal level is under 3 (0-3). You can have your blood tested before you change your food habits. Let's say your test shows your level is 7. First stop eating flour and sodas and take a supplement of fish oil. Then have another test and you will be happy to have a CRP result of let's say a 2. At a 7 level of CRP, you were going in the direction of heart attack, dementia, and disease. But with a CRP level of 2, the bad inflammation is stopped and you will enjoy life much more.

When the brain cells are in a state of chronic inflammation, the brain cannot work at an optimum level. The symptoms are fatigue, lack of concentration, low memory, and less desire to learn. This is happening to a lot of people around us at any age. Some fit people at 50 years of age have a better work and brain capacity than those of people a lot younger.

Dementia is diagnosed when brain deficiency is severe but I think that there are a lot of lower and medium levels of dementia out there.

Bad nutrition is the first cause of brain dysfunction! Now that you know, the ball, or I should say the potato, is in your court!

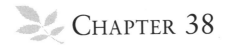

CHAPTER 38

Breast Cancer

Women are more at risk of dying of colon cancer, but are more afraid of breast cancer. I am very concerned with breast cancer. The reason is there are a lot of studies on breast cancer prevention and treatment, but they are not revealed to the public. So all the public hears is "Give money for research and get a mammogram (or other diagnosis test)." For prevention, the public is told to stay thin and avoid alcohol. There is a lot, lot more that is known about prevention and treatment.

Some factors that will help reduce the incidence of breast cancer:

Vitamin D3 in dosage of 2000-5000 international units per day reduced breast cancer occurrence by 50%, and in one study by 85%.

Selenium and zinc deficiency increases breast cancer risks. So supplements of selenium (100 mcg/day) and zinc (20mg/day), will reduce breast cancer risk for those who are deficient.

Iodine deficiency is a cause of breast cancer. So

iodine (1 mg/day) supplements will reduce breast cancer in people who are deficient.

DHEA (DeHydroEpiAndrosterone), an adrenal hormone, is known to protect women from having breast cancer and reduce metastasis (spreading). So DHEA can be measured in the blood, and every woman, if low, can have DHEA optimized with a DHEA supplement (pill).

Estriol (E3) is an estrogen hormone naturally produced in a woman's body and protects against breast cancer. So estriol should be given to women who have hormonal replacement after menopause. Look for research done by Dr. Henry Lemon MD, department of gyneco-oncology, University of Nebraska and Dr. Pentii Siiteri PhD of the California Kaiser Foundation.

Melatonin is a hormone produced in the brain at night and protects against breast cancer and cancers in general. So people who do not dream (a sign of low melatonin) can take a supplement of melatonin (0.5-1.0 mg/nighttime).

Progesterone is a hormone made in the adrenal and in the ovaries and is known to protect against breast cancer. A Johns Hopkins study revealed that women low in progesterone had five times more breast cancer and a ten-fold increase in death rates from all types of cancers when compared to women who had a normal progesterone levels. Progesterone levels can be measured in a blood test during the second part of the menstrual cycle (best time is 17-21 days of cycle), with the first day being the first day of menstruation. So all women who are low in progesterone in the second part of their cycle (after ovulation) are at an increased risk of breast cancer, infertility, insomnia, and even osteoporosis. Progesterone can be given as a supplement in pill form (Prometrium) or in skin cream.

Exercise is known to reduce ALL types of cancer.

Some factors that increase the incidence of breast cancer:

Obesity and insulin resistance are known to increase breast cancer. So a diet with no quickly absorbed glucides (no bread, flour, pasta, rice, potatoes, or sweet liquids) will reduce your risk of breast cancer.

Heavy alcohol use is known to increase esophagus, pharynx, liver, and breast cancer. So alcohol should be consumed in moderation in the form of one glass of red wine per day for a woman.

Provera (medroxy progesterone) is a hormone that was prescribed and is still prescribed to women but was proven to increase breast cancer in a Women's Health Initiative study. In the study, 16,608 postmenopausal women aged 50-79 were given Estrogen (Premarin) and Progestin (Provera) from 1993-1998. The test was stopped after 5.2 years because too much breast cancer increased in the Provera group. No increase in breast cancer in the Premarin (Estrogen) group. Medroxy progesterone (Provera) is not real progesterone. It is not a real bioidentical hormone. Medroxy progesterone (Provera) is a medication that should not be prescribed for the long term. So all women who take Provera should have it changed to Prometrium (real progesterone in a pill) or a progesterone cream.

You see it takes a lot more than a mammogram to protect you from breast cancer. Mammograms help you to survive a breast cancer by providing early diagnosis, but they do not reduce your risk of getting breast cancer.

Now some words on the WHI study (Women Health Initiative). The fear of hormones that come from this study should be explained. This study did not use bioidentical hormones. They used Premarin, a natural hormone obtained from pregnant horses and Provera (medroxy progesterone), a molecule designed by pharmaceutical companies. This molecule does not exist in the nature. It is foreign to the body, as are most patented medications.

The study proved that Premarin (horse estrogen) is good for reducing: colon cancer, Alzheimer's, and dementia. But Premarin does increase the risk of stroke and heart attacks and does not increase nor reduce the risk of breast cancer. The WHI also proved that Provera increases the risk of breast cancer.

So my reading of that WHI study is the only hormone that was proven to increase breast cancer was Provera. This not a bioidentical hormone and it should be banned because we have bioidentical hormones, similar to what the body makes, that can be used instead of Provera. And the bioidenticals show no sign of increasing the cancer risk.

Premarin is good for preventing colon cancer and dementia. But the problem is that it increases the risk of strokes and heart attacks. I believe this is because the Premarin is taken by mouth, then goes through the liver first and increases the coagulation factors that provoke more blood clots in the brain (strokes) and in the coronary vessels (heart attacks).

I think this would be avoided if the estrogens (Premarin or bioidentical Estradiol Estriol) were given as a cream. This would bypass the liver because it is absorbed through the skin.

As to the fear of hormones and cancer, I think the body functions better with an optimal level of its own hormones. For prevention of breast cancer, an optimal level of hormones is always better, mainly progesterone, estriol and DHEA, because they have been proven to decrease the risk of breast cancer when given to women with deficient levels.

The message to take home is:

• Supplements—by taking these supplements, you can reduce your risk of breast cancer by at least 50%: vitamin D3 (2000-5000 iu/ day); selenium (100 mcg/ day); zinc (20 mg/day); and iodine (1 mg/day).

• Stay thin by avoiding foods that make high insulin secretion. No sugar, no sweet liquids, no flour, bread, cereals or pasta.

• Avoid heavy alcohol use. Drink (at the most) one glass of red wine per day.

- Be sure that your doctor checks your level of DHEA (anytime) and Progesterone (in the second part of cycle) and have it corrected by supplementation at optimum levels.

- When taking hormonal replacements after menopause, it is better to absorb bioidenticals (same as women's bodies make) through the skin as a cream and be sure to include Estriol (a mix of 20% Estradiol + 80% Estriol made by compound pharmacies called Biest).

- Melatonin in a low dosage of 0.5-1.0 mg/night can be taken for those who do not dream much. If you take too much, you will wake up early.

- Exercise is good for cardiovascular disease, strokes, diabetes, general well being, stress, and all cancers.

All the money that is going into research does not seem to bring results—the number of breast cancers is still increasing! If some money would be spent on spreading the word about what is already known on prevention, the breast cancer incidence could and would be reduced significantly. My guess is a reduction of a minimum of 50% with the supplements only (vitamin D3, selenium, zinc, iodine). Imagine all the suffering that would be avoided!

For those who already have breast cancer, the therapy of chemotherapy plus or minus radiation is good for treatment but would certainly not be the best prevention. Who would go through a little chemotherapy to prevent breast cancer? The best prevention would also be the best cure. All this information on the prevention of breast cancer can also be applied to the treatment. That means that preventative measures help the treatment.

When someone develops breast cancer, the risk of developing a second one is high, so the prevention of a second cancer should begin immediately.

When fighting a cancer, the immune system is part of the team (doctor-patient-immune system). All the preventative actions are good for the immune system, including bioidentical hormonal replacement. Even with non-bioidentical hormonal replacement (Premarin and Provera), it has not been proven to change the overall survival outcome. I think that with real progesterone, estriol and DHEA, that have been proven to protect against breast cancer, bioidentical hormonal replacement is probably safe. We need a study to prove this statement. So the decision on whether to take hormonal replacement (bioidentical—my preference) is the patient's.

You see there is a lot more to learn, but if we apply what we already know about prevention, much of the suffering can be avoided!

CHAPTER 39

Bioidentical Hormones

Would you put canola oil in your car engine? Maybe canola oil has some advantages, such as a better smell, but it will have side effects too, including wearing out the engine more quickly. A human body has hormones that are produced by glands—pituitary, ovaries, testicles, adrenal, pancreas, etc. All hormones have to bind to a receptor to do their work in the body. The liver will take those hormones (bioidenticals) out of the body quickly, so the effect will not last long. That is the way of nature.

The name we use to identify the exact same hormone as the body produces is "bioidentical." These include testosterone, estradiol, estriol, progesterone, insulin, cortisol, DHEA, melatonin, thyroid, etc. The non-bioidenticals, Ethinyl Estradiol, medroxyprogesterone and other progestatives, are not real progesterone or conjugated estrogen, but they are molecules. These molecules are different from those your body makes. They can bind to a receptor since they are different and the effect on the receptor will be different. The liver will take out the non-bioidentical hormones with more difficulty so they accumulate in the body.

So why are non-bioidentical hormones prescribed by doctors? In the short term, non-bioidenticals can have an advantage because they last longer in the body and can be more powerful. But in the long term, the side effects that come with the patented non-bioidentical hormones will dominate the picture—meaning there are more disadvantages than advantages.

One example of the long-term side effects is with "Ethinyl Estradiol," a molecule foreign to the body that can bind to an estrogen receptor in the body and mimic the effects of real "Estradiol," the real bioidentical hormone. Ethinyl Estradiol is used in many birth control pills.

Observed adverse effects of Ethinyl Estradiol on blood vessels are:

Thickening of the inner wall (intima) of arteries and veins in animals and humans. This is bad for the blood vessels.

Increase in the lipids, triglycerides and very low-density lipoproteins (VLDL). This is bad for blood vessel inflammation.

Increase in blood pressure, which is not good.

Increase in blood viscosity and blood platelets aggregation, which leads to more blood clots.

Decrease of anti-thrombin 3 (a reducing coagulation

substance). Anti-thrombin 3 is a good substance that protects us from blood clots. Anything that reduces it will increase blood clotting in the blood vessels.

All those side effects will not happen overnight. It takes time and they can happen with some people, but not everyone. I think the increase in blood clots from birth control pills is because it is a pill that goes through the liver first and then increases the coagulation and inflammation, which was proven in the Women's Health Initiative study. The hormone Premarin (made from horse estrogen) was proven to increase strokes and heart attacks—two blood clot diseases.

Why don't doctors prescribe bioidenticals birth control? Because it does not exist. Some studies have been done with using melatonin for birth control with bad results. I do not know of any study for contraception with bioidentical estrogen (estradiol + estriol), progesterone, and testosterone.

Why did I say testosterone? Because, when you give a hormone preparation to a woman to stop her ovulation, all that is needed for contraception is progesterone. The ovaries will react like they do with a pregnancy and menstruation will stop. So with birth control, we add some estrogen so the woman will still have periods, but we forget that less testosterone, progesterone and estriol will be produced by the ovaries and that testosterone, progesterone, and estriol protect against breast cancer.

Theoretically, when you reduce testosterone, progesterone, and estriol in a woman, the risk of breast cancer increases because you create estrogen dominance in the receptors.

A study on bioidentical hormones for birth control (estradiol, estriol, progesterone, and testosterone) taken as a vaginal or vulvar cream (to avoid the first passage to the liver) should be done for the good of women. This preparation, bioidentical total ovary hormonal replacement for contraception, given transmucosal, will have the theoretical advantage of reducing blood clots and breast cancer. You see birth control pills are a kind of non-bioidentical hormone replacement system. This is not because of a deficiency, but for contraception.

Any molecule given to a human body should be done respectfully with the best scientific research.

Now let's look at bioidentical hormone replacement used because of a deficiency. Hormonal deficiency should be diagnosed, meaning there is a line, a hormone level measure, that, when lower, is considered a hormone deficiency. That's where not everybody agrees. Some consider it normal that when we age our hormone levels get lower. That is what is considered normal aging. Some say when there is a symptom of a low hormone, even if the blood level is borderline, this is considered a deficiency.

My point of view is:

The optimum level of a hormone is when our body is at

its best. This means a little over the average blood level (lower upper third) of the normal 25 year old.

It is time to take a hormonal replacement when the symptoms of a low hormone (checked by blood test) start to bother you because of the symptoms—usually when 50% of optimal level is lost.

A deficiency is when hormones are not at optimum levels and you have symptoms of that deficiency. The symptoms of hormone deficiencies can be found on the Internet as questionnaires for any hormone. For example, with testosterone deficiencies, there are 10 questions and if you have more than five "yes" answers, it is recommended you have your testosterone tested.

The hormones that can be replaced with bioidenticals are:

Thyroid: (thyroid hormone as a mix of T4+ T3) pig extract (Armour or other). Synthroid is bioidentical T4 but only 33% of patients find relief of their symptoms. With a mix of T4 80% + T3 20% (pig extract), it is more like what the thyroid gland makes and most patients find improvement of their symptoms of hypothyroidism (see the thyroid chapter).

Pituitary: **Human growth hormone,** only the bioidentical is available in the market (which is good).

Adrenals: **Cortisone** (hydrocortisone is the bioidentical), but the non-bioidentical Prednisone or Medrol can have advantages over the bioidentical. This is an exception where the non-bioidentical can have an advantage over the real thing. **DHEA** is also a bioidentical hormone that can be taken by mouth.

Ovaries: **Estrogen** (estradiol and estriol are bioidenticals) should not be taken by the mouth. It is better in a transdermal cream (estrogen patch or compounded cream). Estriol is only in compounded cream.

Progesterone (progesterone is the bioidentical) can be taken by mouth in a pill called Prometrium or in a transdermal cream of progesterone from a compound pharmacy.

Testicles: **Testosterone** (a bioidentical that cannot be taken by mouth) works in a transdermal cream or injection. I prefer injection because the testosterone in the cream is absorbed in the body by only 20%. In that case, 80% stays on the skin and can be transferred to anybody who touches your skin.

The testosterone injection can be given subcutaneously in the fat under the skin, twice per week. Thus, the dose you give is the dose you get. It is a lot cheaper and you will not contaminate anyone.

Bioidenticals cannot be patented because they already exist in your body. The pharmaceutical industry does its best to find molecules they can patent. These molecules perform hormone-like functions in our bodies but they are not the real thing. Until now, patented molecules (foreign to the body molecules) are not superior to the bioidenticals—the same hormones molecules that your body makes.

This does not mean that bioidentical hormones are

completely safe. Hormones work in harmony with other hormones so, before taking hormone supplements, be sure your doctor is well trained in hormone physiology. For example, testosterone given to an overweight patient has a tendency to change inside the patient's fat cells into estradiol (estrogen). This is not the goal—to increase estrogen in a man because it increases inflammation. So the chemical reaction that happens in the fat cells (aromatisation) of that patient can be monitored by blood tests and, if needed, can be reduced by a medication (Arimidex or others).

Hormonal replacement is not easy medicine. It is only for the most dedicated patients and doctors.

Some say that anyone with even one hormone that is low, would benefit from hormonal replacement to reduce the aging complications of low hormones.

Not all hormones are controlled by the doctor. For example, insulin (the aging hormone) has to be kept low by not eating any quickly absorbed glucides (sugar, starch). This is part of the patient's responsibility.

If you are looking for results, bioidentical hormone replacement is a treatment that brings more results than the patient asked for. It's difficult to believe, but I have seen it.

When we prescribe hormonal replacement, it is important to use the optimal physiological dose, no less than what is needed for relief of symptoms and no more than the optimal daily secretion of a healthy 25 year old.

Hormone replacement is not "body building." We prescribe hormones to people who have a deficiency in a physiologic dose—the optimum for a young adult. The goal of hormonal replacement is to prevent premature aging and other health problems caused by hormonal deficiencies, even mild ones.

CHAPTER 40

Fibromyalgia

The name explains the problem—pain in the fibrous and muscular tissues. Fibromyalgia is usually chronic, with a spectrum of symptoms. These include: musculoskeletal pain; fatigue; bad sleep; depression; headaches; irritable bowel syndrome; dysmenorrhea; difficulty concentrating; anxiety; non-cardiac chest pain; and, hypersensitivity to various stimuli such as noise, odors, bright lights, and touch. That's a lot of symptoms for only one disease.

I think fibromyalgia is difficult to treat because the causes are many and all the causes should be addressed to ensure a complete resolution of symptoms. The symptoms lead to a clue about the causes.

Fibromyalgia is associated with irritable bowel syndrome. Most of the time, the cause is a food allergy or intolerance. This is frequently an allergy to flour (bread, pasta, cereals), dairy products, or sometimes corn, eggs, citrus fruit, coffee, tea, alcohol, and food additives. So a diet that eliminates those foods should be started.

Also in the food category, the AGE (Advance Glycation End Products) that are produced by cooking food at high temperatures are known to be high in muscles biopsies of fibromyalgic patients. All food should be cooked at low temperatures—below 250 F or 110 C. Slow cookers or crock pots are very good for this.

Fatigue: Most of the time, the cause of fatigue is adrenal insufficiency. The two hormones involved are DHEA and cortisol. So those two hormones should be measured in the blood of every fibromyalgic patient. If levels are not optimal (midrange of the normal 25 year old), they should be replaced—taken as a supplement in pills. DHEA is available over the counter. Cortisone is available by a doctor's prescription and you have to find a doctor who knows about adrenal insufficiency and borderline adrenal insufficiency.

Dysmenorrhea (painful periods) and headaches: One of the causes of dysmenorrhea and headaches is magnesium deficiency. So every fibromyalgic patient should take a supplement of magnesium in the form of magnesium citrate 300 mg/nighttime.

Other things that have helped fibromyalgia include vitamin D3:

Vitamin D should be at optimum levels for all fibromyalgic patients. This means that by taking a vitamin D3 supplement of 2000-5000 international units/day you can maintain your blood level of 25 (OH vitamin D) at optimum levels, the upper third of the normal level.

The normal range is 50-80 ng/ml. Optimum is between 70-80 ng/ml. The normal international range is 75-250 nmol/L with an optimum between 190-250 nmol/L.

Vitamin B: All the vitamin B complex are important for the Krebs cycle to produce energy in the mitochondria (the powerhouses of the cells). So take a supplement of B complex vitamins. Vitamin B cannot accumulate in the body, which means it is safe to take vitamin B at a higher dosage than what is considered normal nutrition.

Thyroid gland function: Thyroid function is important for everybody and I recommend fibromyalgic patients have their thyroid hormones checked to be sure they are at optimum levels—TSH under 3; free T3 in the middle of the normal range. Those are numbers that you should learn to discuss with your doctor in your diagnosis and treatment.

I think the condition of most patients suffering from fibromyalgia can be improved when treated for the causes of the condition.

Some of the causes are: food allergies; adrenal insufficiency; magnesium deficiency; vitamin D3 deficiency; vitamin B resistance (some people need more than physiologic doses to feel better) or vitamin B deficiency; and non-optimal thyroid function.

By doing what is recommended in this chapter, I think most people suffering from fibromyalgia will be satisfied. This includes:

Stop eating flour, cereals, pasta, and dairy products

and cook food at low temperatures in a slow cooker or crock pot.

Have your adrenal gland levels checked by your doctor (blood test of DHEA and cortisol). They should be in the mid-range of a normal 25 year old. If they are not, find a doctor who knows about hormonal replacement.

Take magnesium supplements (magnesium citrate 300mg/nightime).

Take vitamin B complex supplements.

Have your thyroid function checked and optimized (if needed) by your doctor (Tsh under 3) (Free T3 in the mid range of normal).

You can find doctors near you who know about hormonal replacements on websites such as the Life Extension Foundation (www.lef.org); the American College for Advancement in Medicine (acam.org); or the American Academy of Anti-Aging Medicine (www. WorldHealth.net).

CHAPTER 41

Chronic Fatigue (Syndrome)

Are you tired now at this moment? If the answer is yes, then why are you tired? The chronic fatigue patient is tired for more than six month and since it is a syndrome, the person has other symptoms as well. These include: impaired short-term memory or concentration; sore throat; tender lymph nodes; muscles and joint pain; headaches; sleep problems; and post-exercise malaise.

So the chronic fatigue patient feels tired all the time, even in the morning—even before doing anything. Also, they feel more tired after exercising, when normally the endorphins and cortisol, hormones that are normally secreted after exercise, make us feel good.

We need cortisol to feel good in the morning. It is usually secreted in the morning and peaks after 30 minutes of standing up. The other peak is around 3 pm. Without that cortisol peak, we would not feel good and that means tiredness and all the other symptoms of the chronic fatigue patient.

225

I believe chronic fatigue is caused by a deficiency in the hormone "cortisol." A severe deficiency of cortisol is called "Addison's Disease" and is easily diagnosed by doctors. But there are a lot of patients with borderline low cortisol who have the symptoms of chronic fatigue. They are diagnosed with chronic fatigue without looking for the cause, which is a borderline cortisol deficiency.

But why is there a cortisol deficiency? Your body lacks cortisol if it spends too much of it in your intestines fighting a food allergy, or if your adrenal gland cannot make enough and often both scenarios are the cause.

Then how do you treat chronic fatigue? Food allergies are probably the basic cause of the problem. The most common offenders are sugar, wheat, flour, corn, rice, dairy products, tomatoes, and pineapples. So you must stop consuming all sugar (mostly the liquid) and all flours (bread, pasta, cereal). The first week may be difficult because weaning symptoms will make you feel worse at the beginning (4-5 days) but, if you feel better after the weaning period, that's a win. If you see no difference, then you do not have an intolerance to those foods.

Other supplements that can help are:

Magnesium citrate (300 mg/nighttime)
Vitamin B complex (1 pill/day)
Vitamin D3 (2000-5000 international units/day)
You can find a doctor near you who knows about hormone replacement on the web sites of the Life Extension Foundation (www.lef.org) or American College for

Advancement in Medicine (www.acam.org). The doctor should check your level of adrenal hormones (DHEA and cortisol). They should be at least in the upper mid range of the normal range. That means any result in the lower 50% of the normal range should be considered low. Hormonal replacement of those hormones should be done to obtain a blood level in the upper third of the normal range for DHEA and cortisol.

Adrenal hormonal replacement is done by prescribing:

DHEA in a pill:
Women, 5-25 mg/day and men 25-50 mg/day.

Hydrocortisone in a pill:
Women and men, 10 mg am; 5 mg noon; 5 mg 3 pm.

I am not saying to give more cortisone than the physiologic dose. I'm saying that patients who have low cortisone levels and have the symptoms of deficiency (chronic fatigue) can receive supplements safely with optimal doses of hydrocortisone. At that dosage, the adrenal gland will not get lazy. It is the reverse that will happen. The adrenal gland's reserve (a measure of adrenal function) will be improved when we supplement an adrenal deficiency patient with a physiological dosage of bioidentical hydrocortisone.

A good reference on cortisone supplementation is the book *Safe Use of Cortisol*, written by endocrinologist Dr. William Jefferies, MD.

Most people think that a measurement of blood hormones in the normal range means your hormones are fine. But it is more complicated than that. In order to work, hormones have to plug into a receptor and the health of that receptor is very important for the hormones to work efficiently. This is why some people do a lot better when their hormones are in the upper third of the normal range (achieved by hormonal replacement), because their receptors are weak or unhealthy or chemically poisoned (by pesticides, heavy metals, etc.) and need a higher hormone level for optimal efficiency.

In the end, what is important is the correction of the patient's symptoms that is achieved by giving the right dosage (not too low, not too high). The lab tests are a guide—not the goal.

Thyroid hormones should be checked too. Optimal is TSH under 3 and free T3 in the upper midrange of the normal range. Thyroid hormone replacement is done by using pig extract desiccated thyroid (Armour or other) with a dosage of 30-150 mg/day. The thyroid extract has better results than Synthroid because thyroid extract contains both of the hormones needed—T3 (the active hormone) and T4 (the reservoir hormone that needs to be transformed into T3 to become active).

When given Synthroid (T4 only hormone), around 60% of patients do not transform enough to T3 and their symptoms of low thyroid do not improve much. For optimal physiology, it is better to optimize all hormones but, for chronic fatigue, low DHEA, cortisol, and thyroid are the ones that are most often the cause of the problem.

Most of the patients will do well with diet and supplements. The hormone supplements are for people who do not improve with diet and supplements alone.

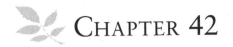

CHAPTER 42

Addictions

CALMING: Alcohol, Benzodiazepine
STIMULANTS: Cocaine, Speed-Gambling
STIMULANTS & CALMING: Opioids,
Narcotics, Tobacco

People who suffer from an addiction are sick and do not function well in society. They are trying to get better when they seek the thing they are addicted to. The goal of the addict is to get better than "The Self," how they feel when sober, but in the end they get a lot of side effects from the substance. The starting point is addicts do not feel good. Then they try to self medicate with addicting substances. The goal is to get better and it does sometimes, but mostly in the beginning.

To understand addictions, we have to look at the brain dysfunction of the people who have a tendency to become addicted.

There are two kinds. The first is the underactive brain, which has a tendency to like stimulants such as caffeine, cocaine, amphetamines, and opiates. The part of the brain that is underactive is the prefrontal cortex (brain region behind the forehead) and the nucleus accumbens (the pleasure and reward system of the brain). To put it simply, these people have a reward deficiency syndrome. They look for happiness, which does not come easily.

The underactive cells of that brain region are dopamine-producing cells.

So the underactivity of those brain cells are not producing enough dopamine, leading the patient into a craving state for more dopamine (the satisfaction, the pleasure neurotransmitter). The stimulants (caffeine, cocaine, amphetamines, and opioids) do increase dopamine.

This sounds like a solution, but the dosage is difficult to adjust and the side effects are huge. In the first place, the action to take a stimulant does not address the cause of why those brain cells are under active in the first place and not producing enough of the neurotransmitter dopamine. Before looking at ways to treat the cause of the underactive brain cells, let's see the other kind of brain dysfunction—the overactive brain.

The overactive brain has a tendency to like calming substances, such as alcohol, benzodiazepine (Valium, Xanax), gambling, and opioids. Opioids please both the under and overactive brain. That is one of the reason they have become very popular with addicts.

In the overactive brain, it is the whole brain that is involved. The neurotransmitters that are produced in higher quantities are dopamine, histamine, glutamate and adrenalin. This leads to an increase in electrical activity in the brain. The symptoms will be insomnia and anxiety up to panic attacks, depending of the level of the dysfunction. That type of person will have a tendency to be anxious and always looking for peace of mind that does not come easily.

So with the help of alcohol or Valium-like medications and also opioids, the patient feels better, but mostly in the beginning. The dosage is difficult to adjust and the weaning effect of those substances just brings more anxiety, so more of the substance (alcohol, Valium or opioids) is needed to have the same effect. No matter what, any substance abuser does not look for the cause of the brain dysfunction that is the reason for the need of a substance or medication.

The causes of the brain dysfunctions are found outside of the brain. They are in the gut (mostly food allergies or intolerances), hormonal deficiencies, and nutritional deficiencies (vitamins and minerals).

We all underestimate the powerful effect a food allergy can have on a human body.

A little physiology:

When a food you are allergic to comes in contact with your gut, it will order a release of cortisol from the adrenal gland. This cortisone will reduce the inflammation in the gut but the part of that cortisone that will go to the brain will be stimulating (feel good). That is the reason you become addicted to that food—the higher energy feeling of cortisol. But the increased need for cortisone every day by eating the allergic food will at some point produce a lack of cortisone in the rest of the body. This will show up as skin rashes (eczema, psoriasis), running nose (inflammation), tiredness (brain dysfunction) and there will never be enough cortisone for the gut, which will be very inflamed. This is called "Leaky Gut Syndrome".

Dr. Alan R. Gaby, MD spent 40 years writing his book *Nutritional Medicine.* In it, we discover that a food allergy is involved in 70% of the chronic diseases and, when allergic to a food, we have a tendency to become addicted to that food. If you are allergic to a food, it is the food that you like the most and you probably eat it every day.

The food allergies and intolerances that are most common are wheat, dairy products, corn, refined sugar, eggs, citrus fruits, coffee, tea, alcohol, and food additives. The easy solution is to stop all these for a month. If a food allergy is the cause of your problem, you will see a big difference in a week.

Hormone deficiencies:

Many hormone deficiencies can cause brain dysfunction. Some were there before the addiction and some came later because of the toxicity of alcohol or bad nutrition. They are: thyroid, cortisol, estrogen (woman), progesterone (woman), testosterone (men and women), DHEA, pregnenolone, melatonin, and growth hormone. To find a doctor near you who knows about hormonal replacement, check the web site of Life Extension (www.lef.org) or the American College for Advancement in Medicine (www.acam.org).

Nutritional deficiencies: Studies on using supplements on addicts have had good significant (better than placebo) results. They are: vitamin B (complex 50 mg/day); magnesium citrate (300 mg twice per day); zinc (20-50 mg/day); vitamin C (1000 mg twice per day); N-Acetylcysteine (600 mg twice per day); L-Glutamine (2-5 grams/day); and, Acetyl-L-Carnitine (1 gram twice per day).

N-Acetylcysteine (600 mg twice per day), has been shown to increase glutamate concentration in the nucleus accumbens (the reward center of the brain). That is the reason why it is a good treatment for cocaine addiction.

Remember the cocaine addict is trying to increase the activity of his nucleus accumbens because of a deficiency of activity and low dopamine in that region of the brain.

The goal of this chapter is to inform readers about the physiology of addictions. Too many people think that stopping the bad behavior will solve the problem. It will help, but the patient will be stuck with his original self. This is where a good doctor will optimize the physiology.

One source of information is www.floridadetox.com. They understand the physiology of addictions.

CHAPTER 43

Depression
(Minor and Major)

Depression is a common condition characterized by a depressed mood, fatigue, insomnia or excessive sleeping, feelings of worthlessness, difficulty concentrating and, at worst, thoughts of suicide. It is a minor problem when symptoms are light and major when symptoms are severe. Some people are lightly depressed for a long time. This is called dysthymia. When I look at the causes of depression, I think that all kinds of depression have many causes and the symptoms can give us a clue to the causes.

Fatigue and low moods are related to low cortisol. It is known that depressed patients have lower cortisol than normal during the day, but higher cortisol than normal at night. Cortisol or cortisone (same) is a hormone produced by the adrenal gland, a hormone-producing gland sitting on top of the kidney. In normal physiology, there is a peak of cortisol 30 minutes after standing up in the morning and another peak around 3 pm and, after that, the cortisone level lowers for the night.

This is important for a strong mood during the day (high cortisol) and for a peaceful evening and night (low cortisol). Depressed patients have lower cortisol than normal during the day so they don't have enough cortisol to be energetic and they have more cortisol than normal at night so they have too much energy at night and have trouble sleeping. This phenomenon is called reverse circadian cycle and it is important in the physiology of depressed patients.

One thing that can be done to correct the circadian cycle (cycle of cortisol) is to take a melatonin supplement before going to bed. Melatonin is a hormone usually produced in the brain. When your eyes see darkness, it produces a shutdown of cortisol release for the night.

The dosage for melatonin is 0.5-1.0 mg at night.

When you expose your eyes to bright light in the morning, melatonin production stops and cortisol is released by the adrenal gland—two good things that help the depressed in the morning. So to be in the dark for long hours during the day reduces cortisol production and this maintains a depressed mood.

A depressed mood is related to low cortisol, so the little things that increase cortisol release by the adrenal gland during the day are good (expose your eyes to bright light) and little things like taking a melatonin supplement at night will help reduced the abnormal high level of cortisol at night for a better sleep.

Those were the little things that can help. But the BIG thing is to take cortisol hormone supplements by patients whose levels have been proven to be lower than optimal by a blood test. The optimum level of cortisol is in the upper third of the normal level.

Signs of cortisol deficiency include: anxiety and memory loss in stressful situations; poor resistance to stress; negativism; feelings of being a victim; excessive emotions (anger, anxiety, panic attacks); and sharp verbal retorts (use of strong dramatized words).

When patients have these symptoms and a blood level of cortisol in the lower third of the normal, I think they will benefit from cortisol supplementation. The usual improvement comes in the first day and, if there is no improvement in the first week, cortisol deficiency was not the cause of the problem.

A good book, *The Safe Uses of Cortisol* by endocrinologist Dr. William Jefferies, MD explains how to safely give cortisone or cortisol (same thing) to patients who have a borderline deficiency by using physiological (optimal) doses of hydrocortisone (same cortisone your body makes) in dosages of 10 mg in the morning, 5 mg at noon and 5 mg at 3 pm. At that dosage, there is no risk of the adrenal gland being sleepy or osteoporosis, a side effect of weaker bones for those who took high dosages of cortisone for a long time.

Note: When taking cortisone suppliments, always take

DHEA suppliments in a dosage of 15-25 mg for women and 25-50 mg for men. This is because taking cortisone suppliments reduces the production of DHEA by the adrenal glands.

One reason doctors are afraid to prescribe cortisone is because of the side effects. When cortisone is given in the proper physiological levels (the perfect dose) to a patient who is deficient, only good things happen.

When adrenal levels are insufficient (low cortisol), the other hormone, DHEA that is made by the adrenal gland, can be low too. It can be easily measured in the blood and the upper third of the normal level of a 25 year old is the optimal level looked for. That level can be attained by a pill supplementation of DHEA (5-25 mg/day for woman) (25-50 mg/day for men). In studies, depressed patients with low DHEA improved when given DHEA.

The other hormones, estrogen (estradiol, estriol), progesterone, testosterone, and even growth hormone, when low, can be the cause of a depression that comes at the age when these hormone get lower (over 45 years of age).

You can find a doctor near you who knows about safe hormonal replacement on the web site of Life Extension (www.lef.org) or the American College for Advancement in Medicine (www.acam.org).

Fatigue and low mood can also be related to low thyroid function. In Dr. Alan Gaby's book, *Nutritional Medicine*, he says that he had 50% of his patients who did improve by treating depression with thyroid hormone supplements. But what is interesting is 85% of those patients who benefited from thyroid supplements had normal laboratory tests for thyroid function. That means, in the depressed patient, there is often a thyroid hormone resistance, which means that those patients benefit when given more thyroid hormone than normal.

This resistance can be explained by lower receptor activity. The receptors for thyroid hormones are in every cell and mitochondria in your body. To have good thyroid function, the right level of thyroid hormone is needed, plus a good sensitivity of the receptors located in the tissues. Those receptors can be poisoned (pesticides, heavy metals, etc.) and less active. That is the reason why a little more thyroid hormone than normal given to the depressed patient can compensate for the lower receptor activity.

This hypothyroid with a normal blood test can be called a hypothyroidism type 2. It is well described in the book *Hypothyroidism Type 2,* by Dr. Mark Star, MD. This is fancy medicine and it works well. The best thyroid hormone replacement for the depressed patient is pig extract desiccated thyroid gland called Armour Thyroid or Thyroid. The dosage is around 30-60 mg per day and the TSH or the blood test for thyroid hormone should be maintained between 0.1-1.0 and Free T3 (another blood test) should be maintained in the lower upper third of the normal range. With that kind of thyroid optimization, the patients who do not respond well to standard treatment have a good chance to get better.

The major cause of adrenal insufficiency (low cortisol, low DHEA) is a food allergy or intolerance and they are: wheat; all cereals and flour; dairy products; sugar; corn; eggs; citrus fruits; coffee; tea; alcohol; and food additives.

So trying to stop consuming these things may help.

The supplements that have been proven to help the depressed are:

• Omega-3 fatty acids. The dosage is EPA 1000 mg/day, DHA 500 mg/day. Read the label. This corresponds to 2-4 capsules/day.

• Vitamin B complex. Dosage 50 mg, 1 pill/day.

I think that all depressed patients should have an optimum blood level of vitamin B12, because low B12 is a reversible (easy to treat) cause of depression. The optimal level of B12 is higher than the lower third of the normal range. Low levels of B vitamins are seen in alcoholics and people with bad nutrition.

• Magnesium. The dosage is magnesium citrate 300 mg/nighttime.

Magnesium deficiency is difficult to diagnose by a blood test because it is the inside of the cells where magnesium is important. Usually, with magnesium deficiency, the patient will have leg pain or cramps at bedtime.

- Zinc. The dosage is 20-50mg/day
- Iron. Iron deficiency happens mostly in babies and menstruating women. It is important to test the blood before taking any supplementation of iron. When somebody has enough iron, to add more is toxic. So only the iron-deficient person should take iron supplements. That means that a multivitamin made for the public in general should never contain iron.
- Vitamin C. The dosage is 1000 mg twice per day. Vitamin C is concentrated in the adrenal gland, so it improves the making of cortisone, which is probably why it helps the depressed and those with the flu or colds.
- Acetyl-L-Carnitine. The dosage is 1000 mg twice per day. This is a molecule that we have in the body. It helps to carry the fatty acids across the membrane of the mitochondria to produce energy. When we get older, we produce less. In a study of elderly depressed patients, Acetyl-L-Carnitine was found to be more effective than a placebo, which is good.
- Vitamin D3. The dosage is 2000-5000 international units/day. Vitamin D3 is very important for many functions in the body, including depression and seasonal depression.

All these supplements have been proven to help. There is also a standard treatment of depression that calls for psychotherapy and antidepressive medication (Selective Serotonin/Norepinephrine-Reuptake Inhibitors). These medications work by increasing the neurotransmitters in the brain and are known to also repair brain atrophy (shrinking parts of the brain) that comes with depression. Your doctor will be familiar with these medications.

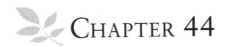

CHAPTER 44

Skin Cancer & Sunscreen

You have been told to protect your skin from the sun because sunburn causes skin cancer. So, if something reduces sunburn, it should reduce skin cancer! The sunscreen lotions have not been proven to reduce skin cancer.

Sunscreen lotions increase your risk of skin cancer.

Some facts:

In the *Journal of the National Cancer Institute*, Volume 91, Issue 15, page 1304-1309, dated June 7, 1999, by P. Authier it states that sunscreen use is associated with increased risk of cutaneous melanoma, increased risk of basal skin cancer, and a higher number of nevi.

In the *Journal of National Cancer Institute* from July 18, 2006, authors P. Authier, J.F. Dore, E. Schieffiers, and U.R. Kleeberg said those who used regular sunscreen compared to no sunscreen at all had 1.5 times the risk of developing a skin melanoma, which is a 50% increase. The ones who used a psoralen sunscreen compared to no sunscreen at all had 2.28 times more risk of developing a skin melanoma.

In *The Lancet* of August 28, 1999, page 723-729, A. Green, G. Williams, R. Neale, V. Hart and D. Leslie reported that in a five-year follow up there was no evidence that long-term use of sunscreen prevented skin cancer. Although in the short term, the efficacy of sunscreen in the prevention of sunburn is undisputed.

So sunscreens do not reduce your risk of skin cancer in the long term. They increase the risk of skin cancer. Sunscreens are proven to reduce sunburn. The whole idea of applying a sunscreen lotion is because sunscreen lotion reduces sunburn, it should logically reduce the cancer that is caused by sunburn. Sunburns cause DNA damage and all cancer is caused by DNA damage.

But things are more complicated than that. When you apply a chemical-containing cream (sunscreen) on your skin and then expose it to the sun, the sun's rays will change the chemical structure (chemical reaction) of those chemicals and will produce free radicals. Those free radicals can cause DNA damage. (*Reference: FEBS Letter, 1997, Page 87-90, R. Dunford, A. Salinard, L. Cai, R.V. Serpone, S. Horikoshi, H. Hidaka, J. Knowland.*) They did a study on titanium oxide and zinc oxide. The sun, by photo oxidation, produces free radicals that lead to DNA damage. These results may be relevant to the overall effects of sunscreen.

That is the reason why sunscreens do not prevent skin cancer. It is because sunscreen protects our skin from sunburn (good), but can cause cancer as well (bad). On balance, sunscreen causes more cancers that it prevents.

Paraben is a chemical found in some sunscreens, underarm products and face or body creams. Paraben is an estrogen mimicker, which means it behaves like an estrogen hormone in your body. This can cause low testosterone in men and low fertility in women. We also do not know what the effect of estrogen mimickers like paraben have on the risk of cancer.

So what should you do to reduce sunburns and skin cancer? First, let's look at the natural ways to reduce sunburn. Sunburning time is the time that it takes sun exposure to cause the skin to burn. The principle idea is the rays of the sun are the insult. The more you have antioxidant and anti-inflammatory levels in your skin, the less you are going to burn.

Sunburn times are affected by:

Fish oil—omega-3 (EPA–DHA up to 10 grams/day). In one study, this did increase the sunburning time by 2 (200%).

Vitamin C—1000 mg twice per day did increase the sunburning time by 21%.

Vitamin D3—(2000-5000 iu/day) did increase the sunburning time significantly.

My recommendations are:

Do not use sunscreen lotion or use it only on exceptional occasions.

Fish oil (4 capsules/day), vitamin C (1 gr twice per day) and vitamin D3 (2000 international units/day) are good supplements to reduce sunburn when exposed to the sun.

Exposing your skin to the sun is a good way to produce vitamin D (from the cholesterol in your skin) and will also boost your cortisone production. Expose your skin to the sun for less than one hour at a time, then stop the exposure before the skin starts to burn.

If you have to stay in the sun for hours, then cover your skin with clothing and a hat.

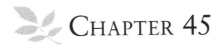 CHAPTER 45

Cardio-Vascular Disease (Arteriosclerosis)

From autopsies done on young soldiers who died in the Vietnam and Korean wars, the blood vessels that feed the heart (coronary) were already damaged in men who were only 19, 20, and 21 years of age.

A vascular disease of all blood vessels, not just the heart, arteriosclerosis is a chronic, slowly progressive arterial disease. It is the most common cause of death in western societies—societies rich enough to have unhealthy diets. Arteriosclerosis kills slowly. Men have their first heart attack at age 45; women at 55. For some, the first sign of the disease is sudden death. The point here is when you are diagnosed with a heart condition at 50 years of age, you've had that disease since you were 20. You were living in a "chronic state of inflammation" in your blood vessels and in your whole body.

So can it be diagnosed at 20 years of age? The answer is yes—by a simple blood test. Can it be prevented? The

249

answer is yes—by stopping all the causes.

Let's look at the risk factors that will give us a clue to the causes.

In the first category are the ones created by food intake. They are:

Hyperlipidemia (bad fat in the blood);

Low HDL and high oxidized LDL;

High triglyceride;

Hypertension (high blood pressure);

Diabetes;

Obesity;

Hyperinsulinemia or insulin resistance (too much insulin in the blood);

Increased levels of C-reactive protein (an indicator of chronic inflammation);

Low omega 3 (EPA, DHA) in the blood;

Low vitamin K (found in greens).

Those risk factors are all related to food intake—a diet based on starch, sugar, trans fat and oxidized fat cooked at high temperatures. It is the sugar (carbohydrates) that causes bad blood lipid profile (low HDL, high triglycerides and small oxidized LDL). It is not the fat that we eat that causes bad blood lipids. Animal fat, omega-3 (fish oil), and omega-9 (olive oil, avocados), cooked at low temperatures, are good. The bad fats are the omega-6 (vegetable oils) in large quantities and any fat cooked at high temperatures (fried or grilled).

The second category of risk factors is related to aging (hormones), behavior (vitamin D), and faulty metabolism (high homocysteine) and they are:

- *Hormones:*
High estrogen (estradiol) and low testosterone in men;
Low estrogen in women;
Low growth hormone in men and women;
- *Behavior:*
Low vitamin D (low exposure to the sun);
Sedentary (lack of exercise);
- *Metabolism:*
High homocycsteine;
High iron.

High homocysteine is an inherited disorder of methylation. When homocysteine is high, it will bring more inflammation throughout the body with more heart attacks and more Alzheimer's disease. The point is, if you test it at the age of 50, it is too late—the damage is already done. Homocysteine should be tested at age 20 to 25 and, if it is high (higher than 7 umol/L), then the patient should be treated with B6 folate and B12 supplements for a lifetime.

High iron is called hemochromatosis, an inherited genetic condition where the body accumulates too much iron. It creates a state of chronic inflammation and premature death. The point is that there are many people who do not have full-blown hemochromatosis.

They have a ferritin level that is higher than 100 ng/l but lower than 350 ng/l and their doctors do not see the importance of reducing their ferritin to under 100 to lower inflammation.

One out of 15 people in North America have a tendency to accumulate too much iron. If you give a multivitamin with iron to the general population, this will cause premature death. Iron is highly toxic when too much is in the body.

The best blood tests to find out if you have an inflammatory blood vessel condition before you have any signs of blockage or obstruction are:

• CRP: C-reactive protein measures the inflammation in your blood vessels. Normal is under 3, optimal is under 1.

• Triglycerides: Tells us how much sugar and starch you eat. Triglycerides should be in the mid range of normal. When triglycerides are normal, this implies that the LDL (bad cholesterol) will not oxidize. This is important.

• Insulin: The best predictive test, insulin should be kept low (in the mid range of the normal).

• Lipids: HDL (High Density Lipoprotein) should be high. To get it higher, stop eating quickly absorbed carbohydrates (sugar, flour, bread, pasta, cereal) and eat more animal fat cooked at low temperatures.

• Ferritin: One of the measures of iron in the body. Optimal is between 50-100 ng/ml.

• Homocysteine: Normal is under 14 umol/L but

optimal is under 7 umol/L.

• Testosterone for men: Optimal is in the upper half of normal levels. Estradiol for men: Optimal is in the lower third of the normal levels.

• Estradiol and estriol for women after menopause: Give enough bioidentical estrogen to maintain FSH (Follicle Stimulating Hormone) around 30 iu/L.

• Growth hormone: Very low growth hormone provokes a state of accelerated arteriosclerosis. One of the reasons is growth hormones maintain the stem cells in our body we need for repair. We ascertain growth hormone levels by measuring IGF-1. The normal range varies between laboratories and also with age. The normal range is 114-492 ug/L and the optimal range for men is 300-350 ug/L; for women it's 230-300 ug/L. It is easy to replace growth hormone when well guided. More information can be found in the chapter on growth hormone, but I consider an IGF-1 under 100 ug/L to be very low and is a cause of accelerated arteriosclerosis.

So, what should you do if you see signs of an active vascular disease:

This is an emergency and you should try to correct all the factors that caused the inflammation in your blood vessels and the rest of your body and brain too. That same inflammation will cause Alzheimer's.

If you do not have signs of inflammation (CRP "C-reactive protein" under 3) that means that you behaved well, but there will always be things to improve.

The best way to treat and prevent arteriosclerosis is:

Maintain a diet that keeps inflammation low. This means eating fish, meat, poultry, eggs (all cooked at low temperatures), vegetables, fruits, nuts, and olive oil. Animal fat (lard) is good if it is cooked at low temperatures. It increases HDL—a good thing. That also means avoiding flour, bread, pasta, rice, potatoes, dairy products, sugar, sweet liquids, desserts, vegetable oils (omega-6), and anything cooked at high temperatures.

Fish oil supplements, EPA 1000 mg/day, DHA 500 mg/day, Multivitamin with enough B vitamin to maintain homocysteine under 7 umol/L, without iron.

Vitamin C 1000 mg twice per day

Vitamin D3 2000-5000 international units/day

Magnesium oxide or citrate 300-500/day

CoQ10 100-300 mg/day

Pomegranate extract is known to be a good anti-inflammatory for blood vessels.

Have your doctor check your hormones (testosterone, estradiol, growth hormone, thyroid).

You can find a doctor near you who knows about hormonal replacement on the web site of Life Extension Foundation (www.lef.org), the American College for Advancement in Medicine (www.acam.org), or the American Academy of Anti-Aging Medicine (www. worldhealth.net).

There is a cause for everything and cardiovascular diseases have causes too. The Occidental way of life did bring the cardiovascular diseases mostly because of fast absorbed glucides (carbohydrates that go quickly from the gut to the bloodstream) and cooking at high temperatures and the lack of essential nutrients. All this is done to achieve the goal of saving time, and then to die early. You can use your time the way you want. What I am proposing is to add life to your time and more time too. Because when you start to eat better, the inflammation in your body will be reduced and every organ will be happy.

CHAPTER 46

Obesity

Obesity is an excess of body fat that prevents optimum physiology. Some people are still healthy even it they have too much fat. But most people who have too much fat live in a chronic state of inflammation. They are tired, do not feel well, have sugar cravings, low energy, do not enjoy life as they could and eating becomes one of their main pleasures.

Most overweight people would like to lose weight, but their main pleasure is the addiction to the foods that cause the fat buildup. So, for the obese, the solution seems to be living a life of sacrifice and be lean, or be big and happy. But what if by eating healthy, you can experience a whole new set of pleasures that you never expected before? This means feeling well most of the time, losing that preoccupation with food, discovering other pleasures in life and enjoying meals like never before.

What are the foods that create obesity? The people who have a tendency to gain weight are intolerant to the quickly absorbed carbohydrates (glucides). They are: all the flours; bread; cereals; pasta; rice; potatoes;

sugar; sweet liquids; and desserts. Quickly absorbed carbohydrates mean they move quickly in the blood from the gut and then need to be taken out of the blood by a spike of insulin so the sugar will be turned into fat in the liver, muscles, and fat cells.

I am saying that if someone stops eating the quickly absorbed carbohydrates, then obesity is gone forever. It is almost as simple as that!

Now you have to learn how to eat, which means learning what human food is.

Human food includes:

Meat, fish, poultry, and eggs. This category contains protein and animal fat, which means they are very good if cooked at low temperatures, below 250 F or 110 C.

Vegetables (legumes). The more diversified the better. They are carbohydrates but in the slowly absorbed category. They get into the blood slowly and do not make any insulin spike.

Nuts. All of them, cooked at low temperatures also.

Oils. The good ones are omega-3 (fish oil) and omega-9 (olive oil).

The oils to cut back on are the omega-6 (vegetable oils).

The obesity problem started when war was declared on fat because of cardiovascular diseases.

The bad fats are:

Any fat that is cooked at high temperatures (higher

than 250 F or 110 C) which becomes trans fat.

Fat made from vegetables (called omega-6). They are not that bad, but should be consumed moderately.

The good fats are:

All the animal fats (lard, etc.). They are very healthy. They increase HDL (good), reduce triglycerides (good) and increase the size of LDL (good). NOTE: All good fat should be cooked at low temperatures (under 250 F or 110 C).

Fat from nuts (cooked at low temperatures too).

Coconut oil is the best for cooking because it better resists turning into a trans fat at higher cooking temperatures.

Fat from avocados and olives (omega-9).

You have to reformat what you think about the fat you should eat if you want to stay lean. The fat you eat does not become fat inside you because it is a difficult biochemical process to make fat inside you from the fat you eat. The easiest way to make fat inside you is from the carbohydrates that you eat.

Since war was declared on fat to get rid of the cardiovascular diseases, there has been little reduction of vascular heart disease. This is because what causes cardiovascular disease is a state of high inflammation caused partly by a diet of trans fat (fat cooked at high temperatures) and quickly absorbed carbohydrates, which maintain high insulin levels and is very inflammatory.

A rich diet of quickly absorbed carbohydrates lowers HDL (bad), raises triglycerides (bad) and makes LDL small and dense (bad). Quickly absorbed carbohydrates are bad for the blood vessels of the heart and other parts of the body.

There is more on the causes of cardiovascular diseases in the chapter on cardiovascular diseases.

The solution to obesity is also the solution to the other diseases that are associated with obesity. These are: cardiovascular hypertension; diabetes; gallbladder disease; non-alcoholic fatty liver; sleep apnea; asthma; stress; incontinence; osteoarthritis; depression; some cancers; and Alzheimer's.

Another way to see it is, to keep inflammation low, insulin has to be low.

The best way to achieve this is to eat more good fats and stop consuming all the quickly absorbed carbohydrates. When you eat fat, it does not create insulin secretion by the pancreas. When you eat sugar or flour, bread, pasta, rice, and potatoes, the spike of sugar in the blood is immediately followed by a spike of insulin (very inflammatory) and one of the best ways the body has found to get rid of that sugar is to make fat out of it—in the liver, muscles, and fat cells. This is very inflammatory (bad) and leads to obesity and other problems.

In 1963, the Inuit were studied. They were found to be lean, with no cardiovascular disease, no dementia brought on with aging and no depression.

With the Inuit, 80% of their food intake was animal fat, mostly raw and uncooked. You see, it is not the "fat" that we eat that makes us sick.

What make us sick is fat and protein cooked at high temperatures and quickly absorbed carbohydrates that provoke high insulin, which changes sugar into fat inside our bodies.

When you stop consuming the quickly absorbed carbohydrates once and for all, (flour, bread, cereal, pasta, rice, potatoes, sweet liquids, all sugars and desserts) there will be weaning symptoms that will last around a week. So you will feel worse at the beginning, but trust me (I am a doctor), after that week a new life will open to you!

These symptoms are a result of the effect on the pancreas, which is used to making a lot of insulin for the high sugar you were consuming. It will take a week for the pancreas to adapt to the new lower need for insulin. During that week, you will have terrible sugar cravings because of the still too high insulin production that provokes very low blood sugar. This is not dangerous. Some people shake and feel terrible, but nobody that I know has fainted.

I did not talk about total calories because I think that it is not important. When you start to eat better (more fat), your brain and all your body will feel much better and you will lose weight at the rate of one to two pounds per week. Advice from my patients who have lost more than 50 pounds: "It is easy when you do not cheat."

CHAPTER 47

Alcoholism

People drink alcohol as a self-medication to treat conditions such as pain, anxiety, moods, shyness, and so on. The problem with alcohol is that it is addictive and with time, you need a higher dosage to obtain the same effect. This alcohol abuse leads to medical problems such as liver disease, psychiatric disorders, cardiomyopathy (heart muscle weakness), immune suppression and more cancer. Alcohol abuse is also the cause of traffic accidents, violent behavior, abuse and neglect of children, and other irresponsible behavior.

Alcoholics have nutritional deficiencies that increase the toxic effect of alcohol and also increase the desire to drink more alcohol. What I am saying is the more you drink alcohol, the more you get sick and then you feel like drinking more to treat the symptoms that the abuse of alcohol is creating. People who have alcohol dependence will experience withdrawal symptoms if they stop drinking alcohol abruptly. These include: sweating; anxiety; depression; nausea; tremors; and, with heavy drinkers, can include hallucinations and seizures.

What is the right dosage of alcohol consumption that is medically acceptable? It is one glass of red wine per day for women and two glasses of red wine per day for men, preferably with a meal.

If you have problems regulating your consumption of alcohol, never drink alcohol two days in a row. So if you drink on Monday, then Tuesday should be without alcohol.

The nutritional deficiencies found in people who drink too much alcohol include: vitamin B1; B6; B12; magnesium; and zinc. Rats fed a diet with those deficiencies have a greater voluntary alcohol intake than the normally fed rats. This is important because many people want to reduce their alcohol consumption, but they need to realize that those nutritional deficiencies keep them sick and always reaching for alcohol.

One of the causes of alcohol craving can be a food allergy or intolerance. These include: sugar; wheat; dairy products; corn; eggs; citrus fruit; coffee; tea; and food additives. So what should you do when you want to control your life and not be controlled by alcohol?

Suggestions include:

If you choose to drink alcohol, the healthy dosage is one glass of red wine per day for women and two glasses of red wine per day for men. If you have a tendency to overdose, then never drink two days in a row.

Take supplements of vitamin B complex (all the B's,

100 mg/day), magnesium citrate (300 mg twice per day) and zinc (20-50 mg/day).

Food allergy or intolerance can be a cause for alcohol craving and other addictive behaviors. If you are allergic to a food, it is usually the one you like the most. So try to limit one of the foods listed above, one per week, to ascertain what you are allergic to.

Adrenal insufficiency (cortisol and DHEA) can be a cause of addictive behavior (craving alcohol).

Find a doctor near you who knows about hormonal deficiencies and replacement on the web sites of the American Academy of Anti-Aging Medicine (www. worldhealth.net), Life Extension (www.lef.org) or the American College for Advancement in Medicine (acam.org).

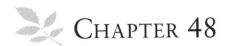

CHAPTER 48

Psoriasis

Psoriasis is a chronic, recurring skin condition characterized by raised inflamed, scaly lesions, covered with a white-gray scale. The causes of psoriasis are known to be: environmental; autoimmune; and genetic. The standard treatments are: cortisone cream; vitamin D analogues; retinoids (vitamin A analogues); phototherapy using uvb-uva rays and strong light exposure; and immunosuppressive medications (Cyclosporine, Methotrexate).

Outside of standard treatment from their doctor, people with psoriasis should learn what can be done in their environment (food supplements, etc.) in order to get the best chance to, at minimum, reduce the symptoms.

Heavy alcohol consumption is associated with increased severity of psoriasis. So by reducing or stopping alcohol, one expects to reduce psoriasis.

Twelve percent of psoriasis patients are allergic to gluten (the protein in cereals, wheat, barley, flour, bread, pasta). There is a blood test to check for gluten allergy (anti gliadin and anti transglutaminase antibodies). If any of those tests are positive, you have a gluten allergy and stopping all sources of gluten in your diet will help you with psoriasis. Other food allergies to look for include chocolate, oranges, lemons, and grapefruit. These are the most frequent but any other food allergy may worsen the psoriasis.

Recommended supplements include: folic acid; omega-3; vitamin D; vitamin B2 (riboflavin); zinc; and vitamin A. All these supplements have studies that say that they improve psoriasis.

Insulin resistance (high blood sugar) is known to be associated with more symptoms of psoriasis. So a diet with no quickly absorbed glucides should improve psoriasis. Then you should avoid all sweet liquids, all flours (cereals, pasta), rice, potatoes, desserts, and sweets.

The psoriasis patient will have a worse condition if, at the same time, they are suffering from hypothyroidism (low thyroid function). So every psoriasis patient should have a thyroid hormone check and even if it is just borderline low, that patient should benefit from thyroid hormone replacement at optimum levels.

My recommendations for the psoriasis patient outside of standard treatment are:
- Reduce or avoid alcohol.
- Reduce or avoid refined sugar and quickly absorbed glucides.
- If allergic to gluten (found in blood tests), then stop gluten completely.

• Take supplements of omega-3 (4 gels/day), vitamin D3 (2000 iu/day), vitamins B (complex, all B vitamins in one pill, 1/day), vitamin A (10,000 iu/day), vitamin C (1 gram twice per day).

• Have your thyroid function checked by a blood test. If not optimum, have your doctor prescribe thyroid hormone supplementation at optimum dosage (for a TSH at around 1 mU/ml). TSH is checked in the blood to optimize the level of thyroid hormone. If you take more thyroid hormone, TSH goes down.

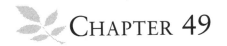 CHAPTER 49

Head Trauma
Traumatic Brain Injury

A head trauma or a stroke can have a serious impact on the functioning of brain cells. Most of the physical, cognitive, emotional, and behavioral effects of brain dysfunction following a head trauma are believed to be caused by temporary or permanent brain cell (neurons) dysfunction. This is true. If we look at the cells involved in the dysfunction, I think we can do something to improve the symptoms and the healing of those damaged cells.

First, the nutritional and supplemental aspects are the beginning of care. A diet that keeps insulin low will keep inflammation low—no sugar, no quickly absorbed glucides, no sweet liquid, no bread, pasta, rice, and no desserts.

Second, supplements that are required for high energy spending brain cells are: vitamin B (complex); vitamin C; vitamin D; magnesium; CoQ10-100 mg/day; and fish oil (omega-3 EPA-DHA).

Cells involved in the brain dysfunction can be all over the brain, but the ones that I am most interested in are the ones that control other body functions. They are the hypothalamus and pituitary gland that produce hormones that have profound effects on many body functions.

The symptoms of brain cell dysfunction following a head trauma or stroke are treatable if caused by a hormonal deficiency after hypothalamus or pituitary damage. The diagnosis of a pituitary dysfunction can be done by blood tests and they are: TSH, Free T4, Free T3 (for thyroid function); free testosterone; estradiol; FSH-LH (for gonadal function); cortisol; DHEA-S; ACTH (for adrenal function); and IGF-1 (for growth hormone measurement).

Many suffering patients have no visible damage on brain scans and their symptoms vary, including: depression; angry outbursts; anxiety; mood swings; memory loss; poor concentration; learning disabilities; sleep problems; weight gain; premature menopause; muscular weakness; and low libido. Many of these patients are tagged as suffering from post-traumatic stress disorder.

These symptoms can be mostly related to the lower hormones produced by the damaged hypothalamic/pituitary brain cells following the head trauma or stroke.

Here are some facts to consider: 50% to 76% of traumatic brain injury victims show some loss of pituitary hormonal function immediately after the brain injury.

Usually more severe trauma leads to more severe hormone deficiency. Hormonal "insufficiency" (level in the low normal range) is seen in patients with mild, traumatic brain injury.

While about 58% of patients recover their normal pituitary function within one year after the trauma, 42% develop more pituitary hormone deficiencies after one year.

The severity of the hormone deficiencies correlates strongly with the symptoms. For example, patients with growth hormone deficiency or insufficiency had significantly worse disability rating scores, greater rates of depression, worse quality of life, lower energy, greater fatigue, and poorer emotional well being compared to brain injury patients with normal growth hormone level.

Restoring the balance of deficient hormones to their pre-injury level has been shown to produce substantial improvement in all facets of traumatic brain injury.

Growth hormone is the most common hormone deficiency or insufficiency in patients with traumatic brain injury at any level of severity. They experience rapid weight gain and have lower levels of other hormones (cortisol, DHEA, thyroid, testosterone, estrogen) as well. Growth hormone is "neuroprotective." This means that, by restoring the growth hormone levels to optimum, it increases the survival of damaged nerve cells and promotes regeneration of nerve tissue.

This way of looking at brain injury is: "A brain cell

dysfunction in the hypothalamic/pituitary that causes a hormonal deficiency or insufficiency, which causes the physical, cognitive, emotional, and behavioral symptoms." For me, this is a revolution! There are around two million patients suffering from head trauma each year in America.

After a head trauma, my recommendations are:

Eat a good diet low in quickly absorbed glucides in order to keep insulin and inflammation low.

Take the supplements that are needed for high energy-spending cells like brain cells. These include: vitamin B complex, 50 mg/day; vitamin C, 1000 mg twice per day; vitamin D, 2000 iu/day; magnesium, 500 mg/day; CoQ10, 100 mg/day; fish oil, 4 gels/day.

Find a doctor who can diagnose and restore the balance of pituitary hormones.

The tests are:

Thyroid function (TSH - Free T3 – Free T4);

Gonadal function (free testosterone—SHBG–Estra-diol–FSH-LH); adrenal function (morning cortisol—-DHEAs); and growth hormone (IGF-1).

Except for TSH, SHBG, FSH, and LH, the optimal level of those hormones should be in the upper half of the normal range. Any result in and under the lower third of the normal range is suspicious and should be correlated with the symptoms of the patients.

Reference: Dr. Mark Gordon, MD, *Traumatic Brain Injury: Hormone Dysfunction Syndrome.*

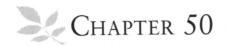

CHAPTER 50

Fatty Liver
Nonalcoholic Fatty Liver
Disease

This condition or disease is usually diagnosed by an ultrasound of the liver (which shows a fatty infiltration in the liver) or by a blood test, which can show an increase in the liver enzymes (AST-ALT).

Fatty liver was known as pre-cirrhosis in alcoholics who drink a lot and have bad nutritional status. Thirty years ago, we did not know that it could happen to the non-alcoholic and now it is the most common liver disease in America. It probably affects one third of the U.S. population, according to statistics published by Dr. Naim Alkhouri and Dr. William Carey, hepatologist at the Cleveland Clinic.

Most diabetic and hypertriglyceride patients suffer from fatty liver. Almost 80% of those affected will not develop liver disease (because of low inflammation), but 20% will develop serious liver disease (because of more inflammation) and that is a large number. The 20% with non-alcoholic fatty liver disease will have serious liver problems that could lead to hepatic fibrosis cirrhosis and cancer of the liver. It is also associated with more cardiovascular diseases and shorter lifespans.

So what happened in those 30 years that caused this liver condition?

The answer is the habit of drinking sweet liquids that contain fructose, sucrose, and sorbitol. Anything that turns into sugar can cause fatty deposits in the liver, but fructose, sucrose, and sorbitol have a tendency to cause more inflammation in the liver and cause a more serious disease.

The fructose that is in fruit is not the problem because the quantity is small and the speed with which it gets in the blood and then in the liver is a lot slower than when you drink sodas. So the liver has no problem dealing with the fructose from fruit. If you eat trans fat and drink fructose, sucrose, and sorbitol, you accelerate the problem in the liver because of more inflammation.

It is easy to see that most of the people who have fatty liver are not diagnosed, so they do not know! If you have been diagnosed, your doctor told you to take care of your diet and you agreed.

It is not the fat that you eat that causes fat deposits in your liver. The fat deposits in the liver are caused by the sugar you eat. The trans fat and all fats cooked at high temperatures cause the inflammation, which makes the problem worse.

The fat deposit in the liver is glycogen. It is not a real fat, but a polymer of sugar. It just looks like fat in the ultrasound, which makes us believe that fat in the diet is the problem. But the truth is, it's the sugar that is to blame for fatty liver problems. Anything that makes inflammation in the liver, such as trans fat or deficiencies in vitamin C and magnesium-omega-3, will make the problem worse in the liver because of more inflammation.

The solution is:

Stop all sweet liquids, mainly those that contain fructose, sucrose, and sorbitol. (All sodas, juices, and even sugar in coffee or tea).

Seriously reduce or stop eating all quickly absorbed carbohydrates, such as desserts, bread, flour, pasta, rice, and potatoes.

Take a supplement of vitamin C (1000 mg twice per day), magnesium (500 mg per day), and fish oil (4 gels per day).

If you do that, fatty liver will be gone or you will never get it!

CHAPTER 51

Osteoporosis (weak bones)

Osteoporosis is a condition that leads to increased risk of bone fractures of the vertebra, hips, and other bones. Osteopenia is the same condition of bone loss but not severe enough to be labeled osteoporosis. One third of American women will have osteoporosis severe enough to suffer a bone fracture. Osteoporosis is seen in men too, but less frequently.

Osteoporosis is also associated with cognitive decline. This can be explained as an organ deficiency. Usually, when you have an organ deficiency, for example the liver, it will only show symptoms in the late stages and you will not notice a problem before it is too late. With osteoporosis, it used to be the same in the late stage, when you have a bone fracture and only then is osteoporosis diagnosed.

But we now have a bone scan test that can ascertain your bone mass at any time and any age, which allows you to monitor your bone health. What is nice is that bone health corresponds with brain health. I believe this is normal because all organs live in the same body and, if one organ is sick, the cause of that sickness is affecting all the other organs as well.

So if we can find the cause of the bone failure, it will also solve the problem of brain failure during aging. We can also maintain the functions of other organs in the body, such as skin elasticity and thickness, kidney, liver, muscles (including the heart), cartilage, fat distribution, and so on. Do you think that I promise too much? The answer is it can be done. This is just basic physiology of how the body works. It is simple—we just have to copy nature.

Osteoporosis is more common than before. In Finland, the incidence of hip fractures increased in women by 60% and in men by 108% between 1970 and 1997. The increase of osteoporosis in modern societies is probably related to change in diet, life style, and environment.

One of the roles of bones is to maintain the blood Ph (acid base equilibrium). When what you eat is acidic (sugar, flour, rice, potatoes), the bones immediately release calcium from the bones to maintain the acid-base equilibrium in the blood. Sugar is acidic and calcium is basic. Ingestion of a large amount of sugar (100 grams of glucose or sucrose) results in a transient increase in urinary calcium excretion, presumably by mobilizing calcium from the bones. A diet rich in vegetables is good for maintaining strong bones and a diet high in sugar will spoil your bones.

In healthy women, bone mass peaks at around age 35,

after which it begins to decline. That decline accelerates for a period of 8 to 10 years at the time of menopause and then continues to decline at a slower rate. If that is what happens with healthy women, imagine the unhealthy.

When bone mass increases until the age of 35, that is when the woman is healthy. She eats well (the Paleolithic diet) with no quickly absorbed glucides.

Her hormones that build bones are at optimum levels and they are estrogen, progesterone, DHEA, testosterone, thyroid, vitamin D (vitamin D is a hormone), and growth hormone. She exercises some. Drinks less than a glass of wine per day. That woman will have a solid bone mass and imagine if we could maintain what is needed to build strong bones—the bone mass will never go down.

In the non-healthy woman, she smokes cigarettes, is sedentary, drinks more than one glass of wine per day, doesn't expose her skin to the sun, has a chronic inflammatory disease like arthritis or celiac disease (intolerance to gluten in flour and cereals), drinks sodas, and may take antacid stomach medication (calcium to be absorbed needs to be in contact with acid in the stomach). This kind of woman will not develop a sufficient bone mass to start with. So sooner or later, if nothing is done to optimize her physiology, osteoporosis will happen and with it, all the other organ dysfunctions including cognitive deficiency.

After the age of 35, all women will lose some bone mass. This is because of:

- Lower hormones the body needs to maintain bone mass and many other organ functions. When 50% of a hormone is lost, compared to the optimum level, symptoms of deficiency of that hormone start to appear. They are: estrogen; progesterone; DHEA; testosterone; thyroid; vitamin D; and growth hormone.
- Nutritional deficiency in minerals and vitamins that are needed for bone health and overall body health. They are: calcium; magnesium; zinc; copper; boron; strontium; phosphorus; manganese; silicon; vitamin D; vitamin K1; vitamin K2; vitamin C; and vitamin B complex.
- Not enough exercise and too much alcohol.
- Possible food allergies. These should be looked for in patients with migraines, mouth ulcers, chronic rhinitis, and asthma. The most frequent food allergies are to gluten (flour and cereal) and casein (milk and dairy).
- Possible heavy metal intoxication. Lead intoxication is known to cause osteoporosis.

My recommendations for everybody before and after the age of 35 are:

- Exercise regularly.
- Avoid sugar, sodas, and eat a Paleolithic diet.
- Take vitamin D supplements (2000-5000 units per day), enough to have your vitamin D 25 OH level in the blood in the upper third of the normal range. When you take enough vitamin D, you do not need calcium

supplements because the calcium in the diet (for example, greens) will be sufficient. 500 mg of calcium per day from the diet is enough when vitamin D is at optimum levels.

• Take supplements of magnesium 300-600 mg/day, vitamin B complex, vitamin C 1000 mg twice/day, zinc 20 mg/day, boron 1-3 mg/day, silicon 1-5 mg/day and strontium 2-6 mg/day.

• Eat green vegetables for calcium and vitamin K.

My recommendations for the those over age 35 is to find a doctor who understands hormone physiology and be sure the level of your hormones, which are needed for bone and general health, are at an optimum level. Those hormones are: estrogen; progesterone; testosterone; DHEA; thyroid; and growth hormone. They are easy to supplement at optimum levels. They all exist in bioidentical forms, meaning the exact same molecule that your body produces naturally.

This is not "body building." We only supplement the hormones that are low and we give the right dosage to obtain a blood level that is in the upper third of the normal range. There are no side effects when we copy nature. The bad reputation of hormones comes from non-bioidentical hormones like molecules that are not like those your body produces.

This is a very important chapter. Bone health equals general health and this for a good cause. I hope it is clear now that the body functions as a whole. That means a good dermatologist could find all the body's deficiencies and diseases just by looking at the skin, if he knows the physiology of every mineral, vitamin, and hormone that is needed for optimum functioning of the human body. He would also know the things that should not be there like lead, mercury, or cadmium because the skin needs the same minerals, vitamins, and hormones as the body's other organs for optimal functioning.

The philosophy of medicine should be to understand the basic functioning of the human body and repair it with what is missing (minerals, vitamins, hormones) or remove what is poison (heavy metal intoxication, bad food, etc.) This is simple basic medicine and it WORKS.

Medications that are molecules foreign to the body are good sometimes, but they do not address the cause of the problem. Medications for osteoporosis such as the biphosphonates (Alandronate and others) have not been proven effective on every patient in the long term and they can even increase the risk of fracture if the patient is taking a cortisone medication or an antacid medication for the stomach at the same time. (Reference: *Drug Safety*, Volume 32, Number 9, September 2009, pages 775-785. Authors: Ing-Lorenzini, Kuntheauy, Desmeules, Jules).

In real medicine, the cause of the problem is what should be searched for to find why the optimal physiology is deregulated. The cause of disease is never a lack of medication.

Osteoporosis (weak bones)

Good nutrition, good lifestyle, supplementation of minerals and vitamins, and supplementation of missing hormones can achieve the goal of reestablishing optimal physiology quite easily.

CHAPTER 52

Migraines

Migraines are painful unilateral headaches that include symptoms such as nausea, vomiting, and photophobia. They are often preceded by an aura, funny visual or neurological symptoms, before the pain begins. Around 10% of Americans suffer from migraines and women are three times more likely to suffer from migraines than men.

The causes of migraines are known to be:

First, there is a constriction (size reduction) of a blood vessel that feeds the head. This has the effect of reducing the blood supplied to that region of the head and provoking the "aura," the symptoms that come before the headache (caused by low blood supplied to those brain cells).

Second, there is a reaction to that low blood supply, including an inflammation and dilatation (increase in size) of the same blood vessels. So the effect is too much blood supplied in a region of the brain, which feels like the heart is pumping in your head—the migraine pain.

What is important to understand is that before the migraine pain starts, there is a constriction of a blood vessel (aura). This is a cramp-like condition of the smooth muscles that are in the wall of that vessel.

Why does a cramp happen in a muscle? It is because the mitochondria (the energy-producing organs inside the cells) do not produce enough energy for those muscles to relax. A muscle needs more energy to relax than contract. When the muscles are very tired (low mitochondria energy), they cramp (contraction). The point here is: if we can optimize the mitochondrial function using simple supplements, the number and intensity of migraines can be reduced.

The second way to look for the causes of migraines can be found in food allergies. Migraines are known to be triggered by some foods, such as chocolate, cheese, citrus fruits, or alcohol. Food allergies include wheat (78%), oranges (65%), eggs (45%), tea (40%), coffee (40%), chocolate (37%), milk (37%), beef (35%), corn (33%), cane sugar (33%), yeast (33%), mushrooms (30%), and peas(28%).

Some of the causes of migraines include:

- The inflammation caused by food allergies or intolerances. In one study, when 60 patients with frequent migraines avoided the offending food, the number of headaches fell from 402 per month to 6 per month, and 85% became headache free.
- The insufficient energy produced in the

mitochondria of the smooth muscles of the blood vessels.

- Low hormones, which are needed for optimal mitochondrial function. In a book by Dr. Sergey Dzugan, MD, PhD, *The Migraine Cure*, he achieved more than an 80% success rate by replacing the missing hormones and giving supplements, without changing the diet.

The solution for migraine sufferers is:

Stop eating the food items that trigger the migraines.

Take supplements that are known to improve mitochondrial function.

Be sure that the hormones, which are needed for optimal functioning of mitochondria, are at their optimum level. These include DHEA, thyroid, pregnenolone, estrogen, progesterone, testosterone, and melatonin.

The supplements that are known to improve mitochondrial function are:

Magnesium Citrate: 300 mg per day
Vitamin B Complex (all the B vitamins): one per day
Coenzyme Q 10: 100 mg per day
Vitamin C: 1000 mg twice per day
Vitamin D3: 2000-5000 units per day
Fish Oil: (EPA 1000 mg/day, DHA 500 mg per day)
Iodine: one mg per day

The hormones that should be checked by your doctor, or a doctor near you who knows about hormonal replacement, are: DHEA; thyroid; pregnenolone; estradiol; progesterone; and testosterone (women and men). These should be supplemented if needed. Melatonin is also known to be low in migraine patients, so a supplement of melatonin 1 mg at night is recommended.

More information can be found at: Life Extension (www.lef.org); ACAM (American College for Advancement in Medicine); and A4M (American Academy of Anti Aging Medicine).

I hope this explanation of the causes and physiology of migraine headaches will help. The normal medications for migraines are useful when the pain is there. They are:

• The serotonin agonists (Triptan, Sumatriptan and others).

• The opioid analgesics (codeine, hydrocodone, and others).

• The non-steroid anti inflammatories (naproxen, diclofenac, ibuprofen).

To prevent recurrences: valproic acid, beta blockers.

Good references books are *The Migraine Cure* by Dr. Sergey Dzugan, MD, PhD., and the chapter on migraine headaches in *Nutritional Medicine,* By Dr. Alan R. Gaby, MD.

CHAPTER 53

Conclusion

Did I start a debate on what is real medicine? No. The debate is already in the minds of people who are interested in their health. Real medicine means understanding the way the human body functions at optimum levels—what all the cells of the body need to be at their optimum.

All the treatments that bring foreign molecules inside your body (medication or natural products) are alternative medicine. This means it may improve the condition, but it does not address the cause because the causes of diseases are never a deficit in a medication.

So I say real medicine means treating the cause of the problem by reestablishing optimum physiology. Alternative medicine tries to improve the symptoms by adding foreign molecules into the body (medications or natural) that do not belong to the body to begin with.

Why have medications (foreign molecules or drugs) become so popular? I think it is because of the antibiotics that were discovered at the beginning of the last century.

Antibiotics are molecules foreign to the body that are used to treat infections caused by bacteria. They did and, still today, do saves the lives of people who would die of a bacterial infection.

So the idea of a molecule foreign to the body saving lives without many side effects is born. This idea (this philosophy) was then extended to other molecules foreign to the body (all the medications or drugs). But antibiotics are only used for a short time (less than two weeks) and the side effects of killing the good bacteria in the intestines can be corrected with probiotics.

It is a different story if you use a medication for the long term. The benefits of the treatment should be weighed against the side effects. If a doctor prescribes a medication (drug, foreign molecule) does it means he is not interested in looking for the cause of the problem? Doctors are very dedicated. They just need to be directed toward the scientific facts of human physiology and away from the "foreign to the body" molecules (medications, drugs) that do not help in the treatment of chronic conditions.

The financial side of caring for the sick has to be considered too. The rule of the game is a molecule that already exists in the body, cannot be patented. So, if you want to make a decent living with molecules for the sick, there is more incentive in developing "foreign to the body" molecules (medications, drugs). Then you have to convince the doctors to prescribe those "foreign to the body" molecules.

I think now doctors are starting to get tired of seeing their chronic patients not improving. Doctors start to be desperate, like I was 15 years ago. The solution is to learn how and why optimal physiology happens and learn how to reestablish the optimal physiology that was lost. This includes a cause such as low hormones, vitamins or minerals, high insulin (diet rich in quickly absorbed glucides), intoxications from heavy metals (mercury, lead, and others) or intoxication from food (sugar or food allergy).

When a patient does get better because the cause of their problem is removed, the doctor feels a lot better too because the best pay for a doctor is to see his patient get well.

I am not against what I call alternative medicine (the medications and natural products that are foreign to the body's molecules). They can help and they are the basis of modern medicine. What I am saying is that real medicine (the medicine of treating the cause of the problem by reestablishing the optimum physiology) should come first in the priority of doctors and patients.

This book is an introduction to the science of real medicine or optimal physiology. I hope to help the ones already comfortable with this way of looking at diseases. I hope to convince those who are looking for solutions. But I do not expect to change the mentality of those who think they already know.

What you think you already know prevents you from learning! In five to ten years from now, everybody will agree with this book because it is basic science. What is said in this book is all documented from references. I only report what I have learned from other doctors and scientists.

Citations:

Merlin Cloutier: "The alternative is to treat the symptom. Real medicine treats the cause."

"The cause of disease is not a deficiency in a medication (drug)."

Writing this book was some adventure. If you want more, tell me and I will write a second.

—*Dr. Pierre Cloutier, MD*

References

Testosterone (men)

Deslypere JP, Vermeulen A. Influence of age on steroid concentrations in skin and striated muscle in women and in cardiace muscle and lung tissue in men. J. Clin Endocrinol Metab. 1985 Oct; 61 (4):648-53.

Deslypere JP, Vermeulen A. Leydig cell function in normal men: efect of age, life-style, residence, diet, and activity. J. Clin Endocrinol metab 1984 Nov; 59(5):955-62.

Morer-Fargas F, Nowakowski H. The urinary excretain of testosterone in males. Acta endocrinol (Copenh). 1965 Jul; 49:443-52.

Gapstur SM, Gann PH, Kopp P, Colangelo L, Longcope C, Liu K. Serum androgen concentrations in young men: a longitudinal analysis of associations with age, obesity, and race. The CARDIA male hormone study. Cancer Epidermiol Biomarkers prev. 2002 Oct;11 (10 Pt 1): 1041-7.

Testosterone (women)

Worboys S, Kotsopoulos D, Teede H, McGrath B, Davis SR. Evidence that parenteral testosterone therapy may improve endotheliu-dependent and independent vasodilation in postmenopausal women already receiving estrogen. J Clin Endocrinol Metab. 2001 Jan;86(1):158-61.

Bernini GP, Moretti A, Sgro M, Argenio GF, Barlascini CO, Cristofani R, Salvetti A. Influence of endogenous adrogens on carotid wall in postmenopausal women. Menopause. 2001 Jan-Feb;8(1):43-50.

Aging

Carnes BA, Olshandky SJ. Evolutionary perspectives on human senescence. Popul Dev Rev. 1993; 19:793-806.

Olshansky SJ. The demography of aging. Geriatric medicine 3rd ed., Springer, 1997, p. 29-30.

McKinlay JB, McKinlay SM. The questionable contribution of medical measures in the decline of mortality I the United States in the twentieth century. Milbank, Q. 1977; 55:405-28.

World Population Prospects, The 1998 Revision, Volume II: Sex and Age. The Population Division.

Hormones

Hertoghe T. 2010. The Hormone Handbook. Luxemburg: International   Medical Books.

Nutrient Therapy

Hertoghe T. 2008. Textbook of Nutrient Therapy. Luxemburg: International   Medical Books.

Life Span & Anti-Aging

Hertoghe T. 2011. Textbook of Lifespan and Anti-Aging Medicine. Luxemburg: International Medical Books.

Arthritis

Pelletier JP, Martel-Pelletier J, Abramson SB, Osteoarthritis, An Infammatory Disease. Vol. 44, 2001, p. 1237-1247.

Caldwell B, Aldington S, Weatherall M. Risk of Cardiovascular Events and   Celecosid. J. R. Soc Med, vol. 99, 2006, p. 132-140.

Obesity

Taubes G. 2011. Why We Get Fat. New York: Alfred A. Knopf.

Bruch H. 1957. The Importance of Overweight. New York: W.W. Norton.

Gladwell M. 1998. The Pima Paradox. The New Yorker, Feb. 2.

Pollan M. 2008. In Defense of Food. New York; Penguin Press.

References

Breast Cancer

Mahmud K. 2008. Keeping aBreast: Ways to Prevent Breast Cancer. New York: trategic Book Publishing.

Chen G, Djuric Z. Cancer Epidemiol Biomarkers Prev. 2002. Dec; 11(12): 1592-6.

Murrell TG. Epidemiological and Biochemical Support For A Theory on The Cause and Prevention of Breast Cancer. Med Hypotheses. 1991. Dec; 36(4):389-96.

Jefcoate CR. Tissue-specific Synthesis and Oxidative Metabolism of Estrogens. J Natl Cancer Inst. Monogf. 2000; (27): 95-112.

Resveratrol

Jang M, Cai L, Udeani GO. Cancer chemopreventive activity of resveratrol, a natural product derived from grapes. Science. 1997 Jan 10;275 (5297):218-20.

Vang P, Ahmad N, Baile C.A. What is new for an old molecule? Systematic review and recommendations on the use of resveratrol.

PLoS One. 2011;6(6):e19881.

Available at: http://www.cdc.gov/nchs/fastats/lcod.htm. Accessed August 31, 2011.

Dolinsky VW, Dyck JR. Calorie restriction and resveratrol in cardiovascular health and disease. Biochim Biophys Acta. 2011 Jul 1.

Iron

Tuomainen TP, Loft S, Nyyssonen K, Punnonen K, Salonen JT, Poulsen HE. Body iron is a contributor to oxidative damage of DNA. Free Radic Res. 2007 Mar;41(3):324-8.

Masini A, Ceccarelli D, Giovannini F, Montosi G, Garut, C, Pietrangelo A. Iron-induced oxidant stress leads to irreversible motochondrial dysfunctions and fibrosis in the liver of chronic iron-dosed gerbils. The effect of silybin. J Bioenerg Biomembr. 2000 Apr;32(2):175-82.

Killilea DW, Atamna H, Liao C, Ames BN. Iron accumulation

during cellular senescence in human fibroblasts in vitro. Antioxid Redox Signal. 2003 Oct;5(5):507-16.

Xu J, Knutson MD, Carter CS, Leeuwenburgh C. Iron accumulation with age, oxidative stress and functional decline. PLoS One. 2008;3(8):e2865.

Cancer

Helzlsouer KJ, Huang HY, Alberg AJ. Association between alpha-tocopherol, gamma-tocopherol, selenium and subsequent prostate cancer. J Natl Cancer Inst. 2000 Dec 20;92(24):2018-23.

Jiang Q, Wong J, Ames BN. Gamma-tocopherol induces apoptosis in   androgen-responsive LNCaP prostate cancer cells via caspase-dependent and independent mechanisms. Ann N Y Acad Sci. 2004. Dec;1031:399-400.

Barve A, Khor TO, Nair S. Gamma-tocopherol-enriched mixed tocopherol diet inhibits prostate carcinogenesis in TRAMP mice. Int J Cancer. 2009 Apr 1;124(7):1693-9.

Jeong NH, Song ES, Lee JM. Plasma carotenoids, retinol and tocopherol levels and the risk of ovarian cancer. Acta Obstet Gynecol Scand. 2009;88(4):457-62.

Iodine

Dasgupta PK, Liu Y, Dyke JV. Iodine nutrition: iodine content of iodized salt in the United States. Environ Sci Technol. 2008 Feb 15;42(4):1315-23.

Gunton JE, Hams G, Fiegert M, McElduff A. Iodine deficiency in ambulatory participants at a Sydney teaching hospital: is Australia truly iodine replete? Med J Aust. 1999 Nov 1;171(9):467-70.

Hoption Cann SA. Hypothesis: dietary iodine intake in the etiology of cardiovascular disease. J Am Coll Nutr. 2006 Feb;25(1):1-11.

Kapil U,. Sharma TD, Singh P, Dwivedi SN, Kaur S. Thirty years of a ban on the sale of noniodized salt: impact on iodine nutrition in children in Himachal Pradesh, India. Food Nutr Bull. 2005 Sep;26(3):255-8.

References

Brain Deterioration With Aging

Bugg JM, Head D. Exercise moderates age-related atrophy of the medial temporal lobe.Neurobiol Aging. 2011 Mar;32(3):506-14.

Alzheimer's Association. 2009 Alzheimer's disease facts and figures. Alzheimer's Dement. 2009 Mary;5(3):234-70.

Pavlovic DM, Pavlovic AM. Mild cognitive impairment. Srp Arh Celok Lek. 2009 Jul-Aug;137(7-8):434-9.

Pike KE, Savage G. Memory profiling in mild cognitive impairment: can we   deterine risk for Alzheimer's disease? J Neuropsychol. 2008 Sept;2(Pt 2):361-72.

Addiction

Available at: http://www.whitehousedrugpolicy.gov/publications/pdf/consdrug_fs.pdf. Accessed April 29, 2011.

Available at: http://online.wsj.com/article/SB100014240527487 0425460457461423073 1506644.html. Accessed April 29, 2011.

Xu J, Kochanek KD, Murphy SL, Tejada-Vera B. Deaths: Final Data for 2007. National Vital Statistics Reports 58/9. Centers for Disease Control and Prevention. National Center for Health Statistics, 2010 May.

Available at: :http//www.oas.samhsa.gov/spotlight/spotlight021counseling.pdf. Accessed April 29, 2011.

Arterial Calcification

Rennenberg RJ, de Leeuw PW, Kessels AG, et al. Calcium scores and matrix Gla protein levels: association with vitamin K status. Eur J Clin Invest. 2010 Apr;40(4):344-9.

Geleijnse JM, Vermeer C, Grobbee DE, et al. Dietary intake of menaquinone is associated with a reduced risk of coronary heart disease: the Rotterdam Study. J Nutr. 2004 Nov;134(11):3100-5.

Schurgers LJ, Dissel PE, Spronk HM, et al. Role of vitamin K and vitamin K-dependent proteins in vascular calcification. Z Kardiol. 2001;90 Suppl 3:57-63.

Kidd PM. Vitamins D and K as pleiotropic nutrients: clinical importance to the skeletal and cardiovascular systems and preliminary evidence for synergy. Altern Med Rev. 2010 Sep;15(3):199-222.

Inflammation and Cancers

Shin SR, Sanchez-Velar N, Sherr DH, Sonenshein GE. 7,12-dimethylbenz(a) anthracene treatment of a c-rel mouse mammary tumor cell line induces epithelial to mesenchymal transition via activation of nuclear factor-kappaB.Cancer Res. 2006 Mar 1;66(5):2570-5.

Renehan AG, Roberts DL, Dive C. Obesity and cancer: pathophysiological and biological mechanisms. Arch Physiol Biochem. 2008 Feb;114(1):71-83.

Enwonwu CO, Meeks VI. Bionutrition and oral cancer in humans. Crit Rev Oral Biol Med. 1995;6(1):5-17.

Liu M, Sakamaki T, Casimiro MC, et al. The canonical NF-kappaB pathway governs mammary tumorigenesis in transgenic mice and tumor stem cell expansion. Cancer Res. 2010 Dec 15;70(24):10464-73.

Food Cooked at High Temperatures

Cross AJ, Sinha R. Meat-related mutagens/carcinogens in the etiology of colorectal cancer. Environmental and Molecular Mutagenesis. 2004;44 (1):44-55.

Jagerstad M, Skog K. Genotoxicity of heat-processed foods. Mutation Research.   2005;574(1-2):156-172.

Sinha R, Rothman N, Mark SD, et al. Lower levels of urinary 2-amino-3, 8-dimethylimidazo[4,5-f]-quinoxaline (MeIQx) in humans with higher CYP1A2 activity. Carcinogenesis. 1995;16(111):2859-2861.

Moonen H, Engels L, Kleinjans J, Kok T. The CYP1A2-164A-->C polymorphism (CYP1A2*1F) is associated with the risk for colorectal adenomas in humans. Cancer Letters. 2005;229(1):25-31.

Wheat - High Insulin & Inflammation

Foster-Powell, Holt SHA, Brand-Miller JC. International table of glycemic index and glycemic load values: 2002. Am J Clin Nutr. 2002;76(1):5-56.

Jenkins DJH, Wolever TM, Taylor RH, et al. Glycemic index of foods: a physiological basis for carbohydrate exchange. Am J Clin Nutr. 1981 Mar;34(3):362-6.

Kloting N, Fasshauer M, Dietrich A, et al. Insulin sensitive obesity. Am J Physiol Endocrinol Metab. 2010 Jun 22.

DeMarco VG, Johnson MS, Whaley-Connell AT, Sowers JR. Cytokine abnormalities in the etiology of the cardiometabolic syndrome. Curr Hypertens Rep. 2010 Apr;12(2):93-8.

Alcohol and Cancer

Available at: http://www.ncbi.nlm.nih.gov/pubmedhealth/ PMH0001940/ Accessed August 21, 2011.

Schutze M, Boeing H, Pischon T, et al. Alcohol attributable burden of incidence   of cancer in eight European countries based on results from prospective cohort study. BMJ. 2011;342:d1584.

Druesne-Pecollo N, Tehard B, Mallet Y, et al. Alcohol and genetic polymorphisms: effect on risk of alcohol-related cancer. Lancet Oncol. 2009 Feb;10(2):173-80.

Juliano C, Cossu M, Rota MT, Satta D, Poggi P, Giunchedi P. Buccal tablets containing cysteine and chlorhexidine for the reduction of acetaldehyde levels in the oral cavity. Drug Dev Ind Pharm. 2011 Mar 31.

Head Trauma

Leal-Cerro A, Flores JM, Rincon M, et al. Prevalence of hypopituitarism and growth hormone deficiency in adults long-term after severe traumatic brain injury. Clin Endocrinol (Oxf). 2005 May;62(5):525-32.

Klose M, Juul A, Struck J, Morgenthaler NG, Kosteljanetz M, Feldt-Rasmussen U. Acute and long-term pituitary insufficiency in traumatic brain injury: a prospective single-center study. Clin Endocrinol (Oxf). 2007 Oct;67 (4):598-606.

Agha A, Rogers B, Mylotte D, et al. Neuroendocrine dysfunction in the acute phase of traumatic brain injury. Clin Endocrinol (Oxf). 2004 May;60 (5):584-91.

Agha A, Rogers B, Sherlock M, et al. Anterior pituitary dysfunction in survivors of traumatic brain injury. J Clin Endocrinol Metab. 2004 Oct;89(10):4929-36.

Fatty Liver

Amarapurkar D, Kamani P, Patel N, et al. Prevalence of non-alcoholic fatty liver disease: population based study. Ann Hepatol. 2007 Jul-Sep;6(3):161-3.

Available at: http://www.cdc.gov/nchs/fastats/overwt.htm. Accessed September 16, 2011.

Koek GH. Treatment of non-alcoholic fatty liver disease. Ned Tijdschr Geneeskd. 2011;155:A3181.

Vernon G, Baranova A, Younossi ZM. Systematic review: the epidemiology and natural history of non-alcoholic fatty liver disease and non-alcoholic steatohepatitis in adults. Aliment Pharmacol Ther. 2011 Aug;34(3):274-85.

Omega 3

Cordain, L., J.B. Miller, S.B. Eaton, N. Mann, S.H. Holt and J. D. Speth. 2000. "Plant-Animal Subsistance Ratios and Micronutrient Energy Estimations in Worldwide Hunter-Gatherer Diets." American Journal of Clinical Nutrition. Mar;71(3):682-92

R. Abe and S. Yamagishi. Cage-Rage System and Carcinogenesis. Curr Pharm Des, Vol 15; 2008:940-945

Index

A

AGE, 67, 68, 170, 222
Advanced Glycation End Product, 42, 67, 68, 170, 222
Alkhouri, Dr. Naim, 275
allergies, 11, 36, 68, 71, 72, 74, 199, 223, 226, 233, 234, 268, 282
Alzheimer's, 23, 68, 69, 99, 143, 169, 170, 189, 197, 199, 200, 208, 251, 253, 260
Ames, Dr. Bruce, 161-164
amino acids, 64
animal fat, 18
anxiety, 187
aphthous ulcers, 71, 188
arrhythmia, 188
arteriosclerosis, 188
Authier, P., 245

B

basal temperature, 94
benzodiazepine, 83, 231, 232
beta blockers, 199, 290
Biest, 126, 129, 135, 210
bile, 17, 40, 41, 139
bioidentical hormones, 90, 127, 128, 133, 208, 213, 214, 216, 219, 283
biphenyl, 69
biphosphonates, 284
birth control pills, 138, 139, 149, 190, 214-216
black tea, 182
blood pressure, 23, 25, 30, 34, 43, 45, 47, 48, 51-54, 57, 78, 79,

94, 100, 123, 124, 141, 193, 197, 199, 214, 250
blood vessels, 11, 23, 25, 34-36, 42, 43, 51-53, 69, 94, 163, 167,
180, 183, 199, 214, 215, 249, 252-254, 260, 287
body hair, 140, 142
bread, 35, 43, 45-48, 54, 58, 62-65, 78, 106, 139, 153, 198, 200,
207, 209, 221, 226, 252, 254, 257, 260, 261, 267, 271, 277
British Medical Journal, 174
bromide, 193, 194
butter, 41, 49, 54

C

cacao, 61
cadmium, 53, 73, 142, 284
calcium, 16, 19-21, 167, 280, 281-283
cancer, 13-15, 23, 43, 46, 68, 69, 79, 95, 99, 104, 117, 125, 127,
129, 133-135, 143-146, 153-161, 163, 164, 174, 176,
183, 185, 186-188, 193, 194, 205-211, 245-247, 260,
263, 276
cancer, bone marrow, 78, 79
cancer, breast, 13, 99, 127, 134, 135, 157-159, 186, 193-195,
205 -211, 215, 216
cancer, colon, 13, 128, 154, 205, 208
cancer, prostate, 13, 145, 146, 186
cancer, skin, 14, 15, 245-247
canola oil, 213
carbohydrates, 11, 25, 45, 48, 63, 78, 153, 162, 250, 252, 255,
257-261, 277
carcinogen, 68
cardiac arrhythmia, 185, 186
cardiomyopathy, 263
cardiovascular system, 141, 143
Carey, Dr. William, 275
carnosine, 169-172
carotenoids, 175
casein, 18, 21, 65, 73, 282
catabolic hormone, 110

catabolic state, 111

cataracts, 169, 171, 174

cereals, 17, 18, 25, 45 , 46, 48, 57, 58, 65, 68, 71, 78, 139, 198, 200, 209, 221, 224, 226, 242, 257, 261, 267, 268, 281

cholesterol, 14, 16, 17, 35, 36, 39, 40-43, 69, 111, 118, 121, 122, 199, 248, 252

cholesterol, high, 40, 111, 118, 121, 157

cholesterol oxide, 67

chronic fatigue, 194, 225, 226, 227, 229

cigarettes, 24, 281

cocaine, 231, 232, 235

coconut oil, 41, 49, 54, 68, 259

codeine, 290

co-enzymes, 29, 162

colic, 72

condoms, 149, 151

coronary heart disease, 51, 189

CoQ10, 29, 167, 254, 271, 274

cortex, 109, 121, 123, 231

cortisol, 91, 97, 99, 109-115, 213, 222, 224-227, 229, 233, 234, 237-240, 242, 265, 272-274

cortisone, 16, 29, 39, 72, 74, 96, 97, 109-114, 117, 119, 120, 194, 217, 222, 227, 233, 234, 237-240, 243, 248, 267, 284

Coumadin, 167

C Reactive Protein, 203

curcumin, 30

Cyanocobalamin, 191, 192

Cyclosporine, 267

cystic fibrosis, 188

cytokine, 28, 34

D

dairy products, 20, 21, 48, 53, 54, 57, 58, 65, 72, 73, 221, 224, 226, 234, 242, 254, 264

DeHydroEpiAndrosterone, 117, 206

dementia, 99, 143, 189, 197-200, 203, 204, 208, 209, 260

depression, 14, 23, 24, 94, 111, 118, 126, 137, 143, 183-186, 189, 221, 237, 240-244, 260, 263, 272, 273

desserts, 33, 43, 46, 48, 62, 65, 78, 200, 254, 258, 261, 268, 271, 277

DHA, 41, 55, 113, 166, 184, 187, 202, 242, 247, 250, 254, 271, 289

DHEA, 16, 29, 39, 91, 109-111, 114, 117-120, 122, 127, 132, 137-140, 180, 194, 200, 201, 206, 209-211, 213, 218, 222, 224, 227, 229, 234, 240, 242, 265, 272, 273, 274, 281-283, 289, 290

diabetes, 25, 26, 33, 45, 47, 48, 68, 78, 79, 141, 143, 154, 164, 170, 180, 188, 190, 197, 210, 250, 260

diastolic blood pressure, 94

diclofenac, 290

diet, 18, 20, 25, 29, 35, 36, 47, 48, 53, 61, 62, 72-75, 87, 106, 113, 154, 156, 159, 163-166, 183-186, 194, 197, 198, 200, 203, 207, 221, 229, 249, 250, 254, 259, 260, 264, 268, 271, 274, 276, 277, 280-283, 289, 293

DNA, 156-159, 161-165, 170, 246

dopamine, 232, 235

docosahexaenoic acid, 184

Dore, J. F., 245

dry skin, 94, 118, 122, 157, 176

dyslipidemia, 143

dysmenorrhea, 188, 221, 222

dyspraxia, 188

dysthymia, 237

Dzugan, Dr. Sergey, 290

E

eczema, 22, 71, 72, 188, 234

eggs, 18, 25, 26, 36, 49, 54, 62, 64, 175, 189, 201, 221, 234, 242, 254, 258, 264, 288

eicosapentaenoic acid, 184

endometrium, 125, 126, 154, 159

endothelium, 23, 34, 51, 53

enuresis, 71

enzymes, 21, 29, 31, 73, 117, 142, 165, 166, 198, 275

EPA, 41, 55, 113, 166, 184, 187, 202, 242, 247, 250, 254, 271, 289

epilepsy, 71

erectile dysfunction, 180

essential fatty acids, 41, 61, 162

estradiol, 16, 91, 117, 125, 126, 129, 135, 137, 147, 201, 209, 210, 213-219, 240, 251-254, 272, 274, 290

estriol, 91, 125, 126, 129, 135, 201, 206, 209-211, 213-218, 240, 253

estrogen, 29, 39, 91, 107, 111, 121, 125-129, 131-135, 140, 147, 153, 154, 157, 159, 194, 200, 206-208, 209, 213-219, 234, 240, 247, 251, 253, 273, 281-283, 289

estrogen dominance, 125, 131, 132, 154

estrogen mimickers, 142, 247

estrogen replacement, 126, 127, 132

estrone, 125, 126

Ethinyl Estradiol, 213, 214

F

fat, 11, 18, 21, 25, 34-36, 39, 41-43, 46-49, 61, 63, 64, 68, 105, 113, 118, 129, 132, 133, 137, 138, 141, 147, 156, 162, 164, 173, 183, 184, 187, 197, 201, 218, 219, 250, 252, 254, 257-261, 276, 277, 280

fatigue, 24, 27, 54, 71, 94, 118, 126, 129, 132, 137, 143, 157, 180, 189, 194, 203, 221, 222, 225-227, 229, 237, 241, 273

fatty acids, 41, 61, 64, 69, 162, 183, 242, 243

fatty liver, 25, 34, 46, 260, 275-277

ferritin, 81-83, 180-182, 198, 252

fiber, 17, 18, 33, 139, 164

fibrinolytic activity, 141

fibrocystic breast disease, 194, 195

fibromyalgia, 194, 221-223

fish, 18, 25, 26, 49, 54, 62-65, 184, 189, 193, 197, 201, 254, 258

fish oil, 18, 48, 55, 61, 128, 166, 184-187, 197, 202, 203, 247,

248, 250, 254, 258, 271, 274, 277, 289
flour, 17, 18, 25, 33, 43, 45-48, 54, 57, 58, 62, 65, 71, 73, 78, 139, 160, 174, 198, 200, 203, 207, 209, 221, 224, 226, 242, 252, 254, 257, 260, 261, 267, 268, 277, 280-282
fludrocortisone, 123
fluoride intoxication, 95
folate, 69, 83, 251
folic acid, 83, 163, 198, 199, 268
food allergies, 11, 36, 71, 74, 87, 223, 226, 233, 234, 268, 282, 288
flax oil seed, 187
free radicals, 157, 158, 246
fructose, 36, 59, 276, 277
fruits, 17, 18, 25-27, 33, 48, 49, 54, 65, 124, 175, 234, 242, 254, 288

G

Gaby, Dr. Alan, 187, 241, 290
gallbladder disease, 71, 260
gamma linoleic acid, 41, 61
gingivitis, 36
glands, 17, 40, 42, 89, 90, 96, 114, 213, 240
Gleason score, 146
glucides, 11, 25, 26, 43, 48, 53, 63, 78, 153, 184, 207, 219, 255, 257, 268, 271, 274, 281, 293
glucocorticoid, 121
gluten, 18, 36, 57, 73, 267, 268, 281, 282
gluten intolerance, 57
glycation, 42, 67, 68, 169-172
glycogen, 34, 277
glycotoxine, 68
goiter, 193, 195
gout, 77-79
gouty arthritis, 77
growth hormone, 29, 91, 99, 103-106, 155, 156, 159, 200-202, 217, 234, 240, 251, 253, 254, 272-274, 281-283

H

H1N1 influenza, 14
Heart, Kris, MN, FPN, RN-C, 113
head trauma, 271, 272, 274
headache, 28, 54, 131, 221, 222, 225, 287, 288, 290
heart attacks, 23, 35, 41, 46, 61, 128, 143, 208, 209, 215, 251
heavy metals, 11, 17, 21, 36, 73, 90, 114, 142, 228, 241, 293
helicobacter pylori, 36, 190
hemochromatosis, 181, 182, 251
hemochromatosis, 179, 180
hepatic-enteric circulation, 17
Hertoghe, Dr. Thierry, 96, 113, 145
high blood pressure, 23, 25, 45, 48, 51-54, 57, 78, 79, 100, 124, 193, 197, 250
high-fructose corn syrup, 36, 59
high temperature cooking, 41, 69, 201
Hipkiss, Dr. Alan R., 169
histamine, 190
homeostasis, 153
homocysteine, 36, 251, 252, 254
hormonal contraception, 150
hormonal replacement, 90, 113, 115, 132, 133, 206, 210, 211, 216, 217, 219, 220, 224, 227, 228, 234, 240, 254, 290
hormones, 11, 16-18, 27-31, 39-42, 74, 89, 90, 91, 94, 97, 101, 104-111, 117, 118, 121, 122, 125-128, 132-135, 140, 142, 147, 149, 151, 153, 156-159, 194, 200, 201, 208, 209, 213, 214, 216-220, 222, 223, 225, 227-229, 240, 241, 251, 253, 254, 272-274, 281-285, 289, 293
hormone deficiency, 90, 103, 216, 273
Hormone Hand Book, The 113, 145
hormone mimickers, 17
Hormone Optimization in Preventive/Regenerative Medicine, 113
hydrocodone, 290
hydrocortisone, 217, 227, 239
hyperactivity, 71, 184
hypercalcemia, 19

hyperinsulinemia, 250
hyperkeratosis, 174, 176
hyperlipidemia, 250
hypertension, 51-54, 188, 250, 260
hyperthyroidism, 51, 93
hypothyroidism type 2, 97, 241
hypertriglyceride, 275
hyperuricemia, 77
hypoadrenalism, 74
hypothalamus, 272
hypothyroidism, 51, 74, 93-97, 157, 194, 199, 217, 241, 268

I

ibuprofen, 290
IgA nephropathy, 188
immune system, 13, 104, 133, 150, 155-159, 189, 211
immunoglobulin E, 72
inflammation, 11, 16, 18, 23, 24, 33-36, 42, 46, 51, 54, 61, 64,
    68, 137, 139, 146, 154, 164, 184, 200, 203, 214, 215, 219,
    233, 234, 249-260, 271, 274-277, 287, 288
inflammatory bowel disease, 71
insomnia, 93, 112, 207, 233, 237
insulin, 11, 23-26, 33-37, 42, 43, 46, 47, 51, 53, 54, 58-62, 77,
    79, 91, 104-106, 113, 139, 141, 153-156, 159, 184, 197,
    198, 200, 207, 209, 213, 219, 250, 252, 258, 259-261, 268,
    271, 274, 293
insulin resistance, 46, 156, 207, 250, 268
interleukin-2 receptors, 157
intrauterine device, 139, 149-151
intestines, 17, 33, 73, 74, 181, 226, 292
Inuit, 184, 197, 201, 260, 261
iodine, 29, 69, 95, 104, 193, 194-196, 205, 206, 209, 210, 289
iron, 31, 55, 81, 82, 166, 173, 174, 179-182, 195, 198, 202, 243,
    251, 252, 254
iron deficiency, 81, 174, 179, 243
irritable bowel syndrome, 71, 221

J

Jefferies, Dr. William, 113, 228, 239
Johns Hopkins School of Hygiene and Public Health, 176
Journal of the National Cancer Institute, 245
junk food, 63

K

kidney diseases, 68
Kleeberg, U.R., 245

L

lactose, 21
Lancet, The, 246
LDL, 35, 36, 39, 42, 43, 61, 250, 252, 259, 260
lead, 53, 73, 142, 199, 282, 284, 293
leaky gut, 74, 234
Lemon, Dr. Henry, 206
L-glutamine supplements, 106
libido, 17, 126, 129, 132, 137, 272
Life Extension magazine, 161
linoleic acids, 61
lipid peroxide, 67, 69
lipofuscin, 170
lipoic acid, 29, 161-164, 167, 202
lipoprotein, 35, 36, 39, 41, 42, 214, 252
lipoprotein, high density, 39, 252
lipoprotein, low density, 35, 39, 42
liver, 17, 25, 34, 39, 40, 41, 42, 46, 111, 122, 126-128, 173-176, 180, 183, 188, 189, 207, 209, 213-216, 258, 260, 263, 275-277, 279, 280
liver disease, 173, 176, 275, 276
lupus, 119
Lyrica, 83

M

MacGregor, Jim, 163

macular degeneration, 174, 187
magnesium, 55, 81-83, 113, 128, 164, 166, 198, 199, 222-226, 235, 242, 254, 264, 265, 271, 274, 277, 282, 283, 289
meat, 18, 25, 26, 43, 58, 59, 64, 182, 189, 190, 201, 254
Maillard Reaction, 67
meat, 49, 54, 258
Medrol, 217
medroxyprogesterone, 127, 134, 213
melatonin, 29, 82, 83, 91, 99-101, 107, 153, 158, 159, 201, 206, 210, 213, 215, 234, 238, 289, 290
menopause, 127, 131-133, 206, 210, 253, 272, 281
mercury, 73, 142, 199, 284, 293
metabolic syndrome, 78, 79, 185
Metformin, 190
Methotrexate, 267
methylation, 251
Methylcobalamin, 191, 192
micronutrients, 162
microwave cooking, 69
migraines, 22, 58, 71, 188, 282, 287-290
Migraine Cure, The 290
milk, 21, 25, 36, 57, 65, 106, 179, 282, 288
minerals, 11, 29, 30, 31, 55, 64, 65, 162-166, 181, 233, 282, 284, 285, 293
mineral steroids, 121
Mirapex, 83
Mirena, 149, 151
mitochondria, 93, 121, 122, 161, 162, 164, 166, 180, 223, 241, 243, 288, 289
monocytes, 157
MSG, 59
myopia, 13, 14

N

N-Acetylcysteine, 235
naproxen, 290

Natto, 163
neurogenesis, 202
Neurontin, 83
New England Journal of Medicine, 174
nitrates, 59
nitric oxide, 34, 51, 53
nucleus accumbens, 232, 235
nutrients, 11, 63, 64, 68, 162, 164, 200, 202, 255
nutrition, 21, 63, 66, 128, 162, 179, 187, 204, 223, 233, 234, 242, 263, 264, 271, 275, 285
nutritional medicine, 234, 241, 290
nuts, 18, 25, 26, 48, 49, 61, 62, 65, 201, 254, 259

O

obesity, 23-26, 45, 46, 48, 62, 78, 94, 106, 141, 144, 164, 194, 207, 257, 258, 260
oils, 29, 41, 65, 165, 184, 200, 250, 254, 258
olive oil, 18, 25, 48, 61, 62, 65, 68, 201, 250, 254, 258
omega-3, 29, 41, 48, 53, 59, 61, 65, 113, 162, 183-187, 247, 250, 258, 268-271, 277
omega-6, 29, 41, 61, 162, 184, 186, 200, 250, 254, 258, 259
omega-9, 41, 48, 61, 65, 201, 250, 258, 259
opioids, 232, 233
osteoarthritis, 68, 260
osteopenia, 279
osteoporosis, 21, 69, 118, 126, 143, 207, 239, 279, 280-284
ovaries, 40, 132, 134, 139, 206, 213, 215
ovulating, 125, 150
oxidation, 35, 42
oxytocin, 157

P

Paleolithic diet, 18, 25, 26, 48, 54, 58, 62, 106, 113, 281, 282
pancreas, 23, 25, 46, 47, 60, 79, 153, 180, 198, 213, 260, 261
pancreatitis, 188
paraben, 247

Parkinson's, 99, 197, 199

pasta, 25, 26, 33, 35, 43-48, 54, 58, 62-65, 71, 78, 139, 153, 198, 200, 207, 209, 221, 224, 226, 252, 254, 257, 260, 261, 267, 268, 271, 277

peripheral vascular disease, 51

pernicious anemia, 190

pesticides, 11, 17, 21, 36, 59, 90, 95, 114, 142, 158, 228, 241

pheromones, 149, 150

photophobia, 287

photosensitivity, 188

phthalate, 69

pineal gland, 99

pituitary gland, 93, 103, 106, 272

plaque, 34-36, 42

pomegranate extract, 202

post-traumatic stress syndrome, 111

potatoes, 25, 26, 33, 35, 43, 45-48, 54, 58, 62, 65, 68, 153, 160, 198, 200, 207, 254, 257, 260, 261, 268, 277, 280

poultry, 25, 26, 49, 54, 62, 64, 254, 258

prednisone, 217

prefrontal cortex, 231

pregnenolone, 16, 39, 91, 109-111, 119-122, 194, 200, 201, 234, 289, 290

pregnenolone steal, 110, 119

Premarin, 127, 128, 207-211, 215

premenopausal, 125, 131, 134, 135, 186

presbitia, 171

preventive medicine, 87

Prilosec, 190

progesterone, 29, 39, 91, 109, 125-135, 153, 154, 159, 194, 200, 201, 206-211, 213-216, 218, 234, 240, 281-283, 289, 290

progestin, 134

Prometrium, 126, 129, 134, 207, 208, 218

proteins, 11, 39, 42, 63, 73, 162, 170

proton, 190

Provera, 127, 134, 207, 208, 211

PSA, 146
psoriasis, 71, 188, 267, 268

R

rast test, 73
Raynaud's disease, 188
reactive hypoglycemia, 71
renal failure, 51
Requip, 83
restless leg syndrome, 81, 82, 180
resveratrol, 30, 202
rheumatoid arthritis, 68, 119, 188
rhinitis, 71, 282
rice, 25, 26, 33, 35, 43, 45-48, 54, 58, 62, 198, 200, 207, 226, 254, 257, 260, 261, 268, 271, 277, 280
Rothenberg, Dr. Ron, 113

S

sarcoidosis, 19
saw palmetto, 30
scratch test, 73
seasonal affective disorder, 100
secretagogue, 106, 107
Selective Serotonin/Norepinephrine-Reuptake Inhibitors, 243
selenium, 29, 95, 104, 166, 195, 202, 205, 209, 210
Shieffiers, E., 245
Siiteri, Dr. Pentii, 206
Sinatra, Dr. Steven, 82
sorbitol, 276, 277
Star, Dr. Mark, 97, 241
statins, 199
stem cells, 90, 91, 105, 106, 155, 253
steroid hormone, 16-18, 39, 40, 42, 111, 113, 117, 119, 121-123, 157, 180, 194
steroid hormone receptors, 194
stevia, 59

stress, 53, 109-115, 118, 119, 140, 210, 239, 260, 272

strokes, 23, 46, 143, 209, 210, 215

sucrose, 276, 277, 280

sugar, 21-26, 31, 33-7, 45-47, 53, 57-62, 64, 65 67, 72, 78, 79, 106, 153, 154, 159, 160, 164, 170, 171, 174, 198, 201, 209, 219, 226, 234, 242, 250, 252, 254, 258, 260, 261, 264, 268, 271, 276, 277, 280, 282, 288, 293

sugar craving, 23, 37, 45, 47, 61, 257, 261

Sumatriptan, 290

sunburn, 15, 245-248

sun exposure, 14, 15, 18, 247

sunscreen lotions, 15, 245

supplements, 13-15, 19, 21, 27-30, 40, 55, 65, 81-83, 87, 95-97, 100, 106, 113, 119-121, 128, 132, 134, 140, 146, 155-158, 162-167, 172, 175-187, 190, 194, 195, 201-206, 209, 210, 219, 224-229, 235, 239, 241-243, 248, 251, 254, 264-269, 271, 274, 282, 283, 288, 289

sympathetic autonomic nervous system, 109

Synthroid, 96, 217, 228

systolic blood pressure, 94

sweet liquids, 25, 33, 43-48, 58, 59, 62-65, 78, 153, 198, 200, 207, 209, 258, 261, 268, 276, 277

T

T3 hormone, 96

T4 hormone, 96

testosterone, 16, 29, 39, 91, 107, 111, 117, 129, 133, 137-147, 150, 151, 194, 200, 201, 213-219, 234, 240, 247, 251-254, 272-274, 281-283, 289, 290

thiamine, 69

thyroid, 27, 29, 40, 55, 74, 91-97, 107, 114, 153, 156, 157, 159, 176, 193, 199-201, 213, 217, 223, 224, 228, 229, 234, 241, 242, 254, 268, 269, 272-274, 281-283, 289, 290

thyroid T3, 99

titanium oxide, 246

tocopherol, 83, 173

tocotrienol, 83, 173
toxins, 21, 36, 53, 67, 68
trans fat, 18, 36, 41-43, 49, 61, 68, 250, 259, 276, 277
triglycerides, 34, 42, 43, 61, 188, 214, 250, 252, 259, 260
Triptan, 290
tuberculosis, 19

U

uric acid, 77-79

V

Valium, 232, 233
valproic acid, 290
vegetables, 17, 18, 20, 25, 26, 48, 49, 54, 62, 64, 139, 200, 254,
    258, 259, 280, 283
vitamins, 11, 29-31, 64-69, 113, 162, 164-166, 173-175, 181,
    198-202, 223, 233, 242, 269, 282, 284, 285, 289, 293
vitamin A, 65, 66, 173-177, 192, 267-269
vitamin B, 165, 166, 223-226, 235, 242, 264, 271
vitamin B12, 69, 189-192, 199, 242
vitamin B complex, 223, 224, 274, 282, 283, 289
vitamin C, 27, 55, 65, 66, 69, 113, 128, 166, 202, 235, 243, 247,
    248, 254, 269, 271, 274, 277, 282, 283, 289
vitamin D, 13-21, 36, 39, 53, 55, 65, 66, 95, 104, 128, 156, 166,
    177, 192, 195, 222, 248, 251, 267, 268, 271, 274, 281-283
vitamin D3, 14, 15, 19, 95, 201, 202, 205, 209, 210, 222, 223,
    226, 243, 247, 248, 254, 269, 289
vitamin E, 83, 173
vitamin K, 163, 165, 167, 250, 283

W

wegener, 119
wheat, 17, 71-73, 226, 234, 242, 264, 267, 288
wine, 106, 207, 209, 264, 281
Women's Health Initiative, 127, 207, 215

X

Xanax, 232
xenobiotic, 36
Xylitol, 60

Y

yogurt, 57, 65, 106

Z

Zantac, 190
zinc, 15, 29, 95, 104, 166, 195, 202, 205, 209, 210, 235, 243, 246, 264, 265, 268, 282, 283
zinc oxide, 246